An Illustrative Guide on Platelet Rich Plasma

Drs. SANDEEP AND
DEEPTI SHRIVASTAVA

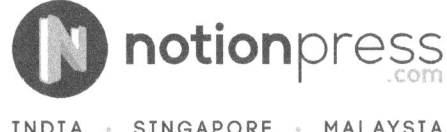

INDIA · SINGAPORE · MALAYSIA

Notion Press

Old No. 38, New No. 6
McNichols Road, Chetpet
Chennai - 600 031

First Published by Notion Press 2019
Copyright © Drs. Sandeep and Deepti Shrisvastava 2019
All Rights Reserved.

ISBN 978-1-64678-611-4

Dedicated

To

"LORD - TIRUPATI"

&

All those who continue to suffer because of lack of resources and limitation of Modern Medicine, with the hopethat adequate solutions will emerge to make them smile again.

Contents

Preface 9

Acknowledgements 11

Chapter I

Basics about PRP

1. Definition... 13

2. Key Evidences for Platelet Concentration & Optimal Stimulation........................ 15

3. Properties of Platelets... 17

4. Clinical Implications of PRP 21

5. Preparation of PRP 23

6. Key Evidences for PRP 33

Chapter II

PRP for Wounds

1. Introduction 37

2. Rationale 38

3.   Key Evidences... 39

4.   Our Experience 41

Chapter III

ATLAS of STARS Therapy

1.   Introduction 45

2.   The Technique 48

3.   The Clinical Protocols... 55

4.   Development & Rationale 58

5.   Problems/Difficulties and Complications... 71

6.   Pathology of Wound Healing by STARS Therapy............................ 72

7.   Illustrated Prototype Cases... 76

Chapter IV

PRP for Tendinopathies

1.   Introduction 89

2.   Rationale 92

3.   Key Evidence in Literature 95

4.   Our Experience 97

Chapter V

PRP in Osteoarthritis of Knee

1.   Introduction 105

2.   Rationale 106

3.   Current Trends.. 107

4. Key Evidences in Literature... 109

5. Our Experience... 111

Chapter VI

PRP for Fracture Impairments5

1. Introduction 117

2. Rationale 118

3. Key Evidence in Literature 120

4. Our Experience 122

Chapter VII

PRP in Subfertility/Infertility

1. Endometrium Regeneration.. 129

2. Ovarian Rejuvenation 134

List of Figures & Tables.. 139

Acknowledgements and Reference for Further Reading 145

About Authors 155

Preface

The advent of regenerative medicine is a paradigm shift from Tissue Repairs to Regenerations.

Platelet-rich Plasma is a key regenerative product based on cellular therapy that has immense potential to induce and propagate tissue regeneration. Its ease of preparedness and bio-safety makes it accessible and affordable product for the clinical applications.

The other key regenerative medicine product such as the Stem cells including Adult Stem cells, Mesenchymal Stem Cells, Bioengineered Stem Cells need huge resource with state of art environment. This is a major challenge for their clinical applications.

The availability and results have opened a huge opportunity to build solutions for many complex health problems and offer better the treatments and prognosis. This includes degenerative diseases, reproductive problems such as IVF, Fracture impairments & tendinopathies etc.

Wounds are also one such health problem. With the increase in violence and Co-Morbidities, the incidences are rising and outcomes not so better.

Over the ages, these have been treated classically by Local care through various dressing materials, which were available in local vicinities like Honey, alcohol, etc.

With the development in sciences particularly related to chemistry and drug development, the role of drugs to prevent and treat infections such as antibiotics; and to control pain such as analgesics got incorporated in the wound management.

As the surgery became safer, intense surgical interventions were developed including for cleaning of wounds such as debridement and irrigation. These were followed by reconstruction such as skin gratings and microvascular flaps.

Later, particularly in the early 21ˢᵗ century, a lot of devices were developed such as negative suction pressure devices to keep the wounds sterile and shrink gradually.

But despite the development and incorporation of these intense management wound healing remains a huge challenge and burden to society.

The Author has developed a clinical protocol (STRAS) based on PRP.

The atlas discusses it in detail, the technique, the indications, contraindications, results of the same.

The results are astonishing and the first-time solution the reversal of Gangrenous/necrotic changes is now possible.

This regenerative therapy based only on PRP is turning to be a "game-changer" and with a single product – healing, control of infection and control of pain is now possible.

We hope by providing visual-based literature on the same, we will be helpful to guide Medical doctors, nursing staff and other health care workers across the globe to undertake it with confidence and bring relief to millions.

Acknowledgements

We acknowledge the support & help rendered by all the Project Coordinators & Assistants at Centre for Regenerative Medicine, including Dr. P. Singh, Dr. C. Mahakalkar, Dr. S. Shukla, Dr. Pankaj Kharabe, Dr. A.Pundkar, Dr. Virul Shrivastava & Sr.Sujata.

We are thankful to all our Professional Colleagues and Postgraduates at Dept. of Orthopaedics, Dept. OF Obstetrics & Gynecology, Wardha test tube Centre and the Hospital Staff at A.V.B. Rural Hospital, Sawangi Wardha.

We will ever remain grateful to our Parents: Late Dr. Pratap Ram Shrivastava & Late Mrs. Urmila Shrivastava, Shri T.S. Khare and Smt. Shakuntala Khare; "They continue to inspire us everyday"

We are extremely thankful to our Siblings and their families:

Rachna & Sanjay, Ranjana & Rajiv, Roopam & Vikas and Rinku & Manish.

Devesh & Garima, Yogesh & Abhilasha.

who supported our endeavor excitedly and kept us going to develop it little by little.

Our special gratitude to our children, Priyal & Prakher, who not only patiently allowed us to prioritize this work but also actively participated in writing few papers along.

"We are so Proud of them."

– Sandeep Shrivastava Deepti Shrivastava

Chapter I

Basics about PRP

1

Definition

Blood = Plasma (55%) + Blood cells (45%).

The human plasma mainly contains Red Blood Cells (RBC); White Blood Cells (WBC) and Platelets.

The normal value of Platelets is variable between 150,000 to 450000 (1.5 to 4 Lacs)/per ml, (average of about 250,000 per mm3).

The Platelet Rich Plasma (PRP) has been defined in many ways.

As per the PubMed – It is a preparation consisting of Platelets concentrated in a limited volume of Plasma. The PRP word was introduced in 2007.

A superfluous concentration of the platelets in plasma is the PRP.

It is a viable and intact concentration of human platelets in a small volume.

The PRP is the platelet concentrate of 3–10 times its normal value.

A therapeutic PRP concentrate should be about 3-8 times of normal value.

The PRP definition is still not fixed, as far as the exact quantity of platelet concentrate is considered.

There are different synonyms used for PRP.

These include Autologous Platelet Concentrate (APC), Autologous conditioned plasma, Platelet Rich Fibrin (PRF)

The MeSH unique ID is D053657.

The PRP/APC are further sub-grouped into 4 general categories based on the leucocyte and fibrin contents, as per Ehrenfest et al (2009), depending on their cell counts and Fibrin architecture.

1. **L-PRP (Leukocyte rich PRP)**: They are with Leucocyte PRP product, without leucocytes and with a low-density fibrin network after activation. They are the commonest one available as commercial kits.

2. **P-PRP (Leucocyte reduced PRP):** They are Leucocyte Poor PRP product, without leucocytes and with a low-density fibrin network after activation.

3. **Leucocyte platelet-rich fibrin (L-PRF):** These are second generation PRP products with leucocytes and with high density fibrin network.

4. **Pure Platelet-rich Fibrin (P-PRF):** They are Leucocyte Poor PRP product, without leucocytes and with a high -density fibrin network after activation. These products exist in a strongly activated gel form, and cannot be injected or used like traditional fibrin glue.

2

Key Evidences for Platelet Concentration & Optimal Stimulation

- **Bowen-Pope et al (1986)** there are approximately 0.06 ng of PDGF per one million platelets.

- **Whitman DH et al (1997),** a platelet count of 1000 x 10^9 platelets/L, as measured in a volume of 5 ml of plasma, may be the **"therapeutic dose" of PRP.**

- **Paques M et al (1999)** demonstrated that 1 mL of platelet (10^9 platelets/ml) contain 115 ng of PDGF, 106 ng of TGF-β, 20.8 ng of FGF, and 0.8 ng of PDEGF.

- **Weibrich et al (2001)** Platelet count in PRP was 5 times higher than the donor blood, – higher concentration of growth factors were found in PRP, platelet concentration or growth factor concentration except for TGF levels which displayed a slight decrease in concentration with age.

- **Weibrich G et al (2004)** suggested that platelet concentrations ranging from 800 to 1200 x 10^9 platelets/μL are necessary to obtain an effective PRP dose.

- **Anitua et al (2004)** stated that the platelet count of **PRP should be more than 3,00,000/μl.**

- **Marx** gave a Platelet count of 10 lakh/ml in 5 mL of PRP, as a working definition of PRP, based on the scientific proof of bone and soft tissue healing enhancement.

- **Rughetti** *et al*:

- Studied the relationship between the concentration of platelets in platelet gel and changes in the functional activity of human endothelial cells.

- The proliferation of endothelial cells and its migration and the invasion of endothelial cells occurred in a bell-shaped manner.

- The stimulation Peaks: Proliferation of endothelial cells at 1.25×10^6 and angiogenesis at 1.5×10^6 platelets/mL, respectively.
- This signifies the fact that a PRP platelet count 1 million/mL has become the working definition for therapeutic PRP

The variability in platelet concentrating techniques alter platelet degranulation characteristics that affect the clinical outcomes. The proponents of PRP therapy have argued that negative clinical results are associated with poor-quality PRP produced by inadequate single spin devices.

3

Properties of Platelets

Platelets: Cytoplasmic fragments of megakaryocytes, formed in the marrow and are approximately 2 μm in diameter

The Fundamental role played by platelet is in haemostasis or tissue healing. They contain more than 30 bioactive protein. They are initiated by secretory Molecules including cytokines, growth factors, coagulation factors, Chemokines, and Integrins. These are all packed in Macrophage vesicles as Granules, Lysomes and Core Dense Granule. In the zymogenic state these are called alpha granules. On disintegrating these alpha granules liberate the growth factors. M. Christgau D. Moder K.-A. Hiller et al in September 2006 published that the APC contained 2.2×106 platelets/μl, which was 7.9 times more than in the venous blood. Transforming growth factor-β1 (TGF-β1), insulin-like growth factor-I (IGF-I), platelet-derived growth factor-AB (PDGF-AB), PDGF-BB, vascular endothelial growth factor (VEGF), and epidermal growth factor (EGF) were found in the APC, whereas interleukin-1β (IL-1β), IL-6, tumor necrosis factor α (TNFα), IL-4, and IL-10 were not detectable.

The role of Key Growth Factors & their primary functions are as per Table no.1.

Growth Factor	Primary Functions
Epidermal Growth Factors	Regulation of cell proliferation, differentiation and survival
Insulin Like Growth Factor	Key regulator of cell metabolism and growth Stimulates proliferation and differentiation functions in osteoblasts
Platelet Derived Growth Factor	Major mitogen for connective tissue cells and certain other cell types. Promotes the synthesis of collagen and structural proteins
Transforming Growth Factors	Regulation of cell Proliferation, Differentiation and Apoptosis Induction of intimal thickening
Vascular Endothelial Growth Factor	Regulation of Angiogenesis

Table No.1: Showing different growth factors and their primary role.

These aids the regeneration through effecting the microenvironment as per table no.2

PDGF-αα, αβ, ββ	Chemotactic for fibroblasts and macrophages
	Mitogenic for fibroblasts, smooth muscle cells and endothelial cells
TGF*- β1, β2	Mediates angiogenesis
	Chemotactic for fibroblasts, keratinocytes and macrophages
	Mitogenic for fibroblasts and smooth muscle cells
	Inhibits endothelial cells, keratinocytes and lymphocytes
	Regulates matrix proteins, including collagen, proteoglycans, fibronectin and matrix-degrading proteins
VEGF†	Chemotactic and mitogenic for endothelial cells
	Mediates angiogenesis
EGF‡	Mediates angiogenesis
	Mitogenic for fibroblasts, endothelial cells and keratinocytes
HGF§	Mediates regeneration
FGF‖	Mediates tissue organization and regeneration
FGF-9	Aids generation of new follicles

Table No.2: Effect of Growth Factors on Microenvironment during tissue regeneration

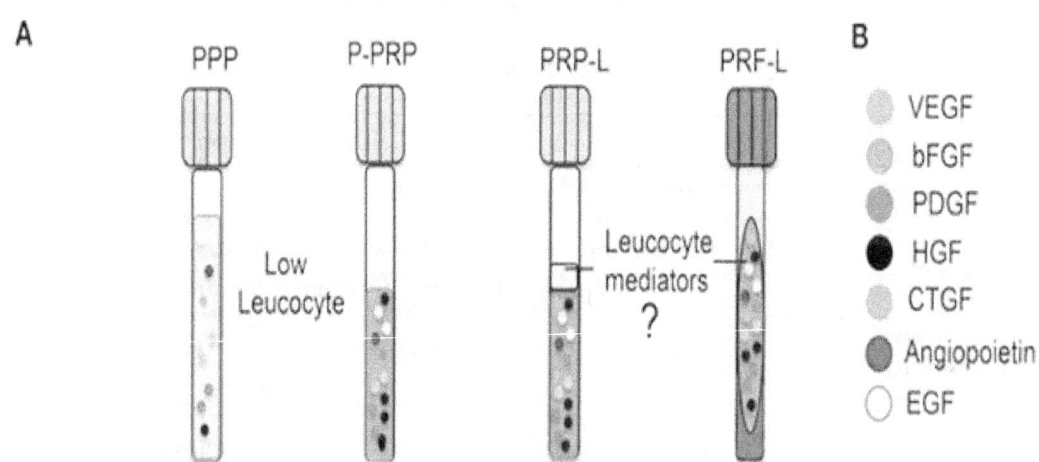

Fig.1: Different PRP preparations and the Growth factors.

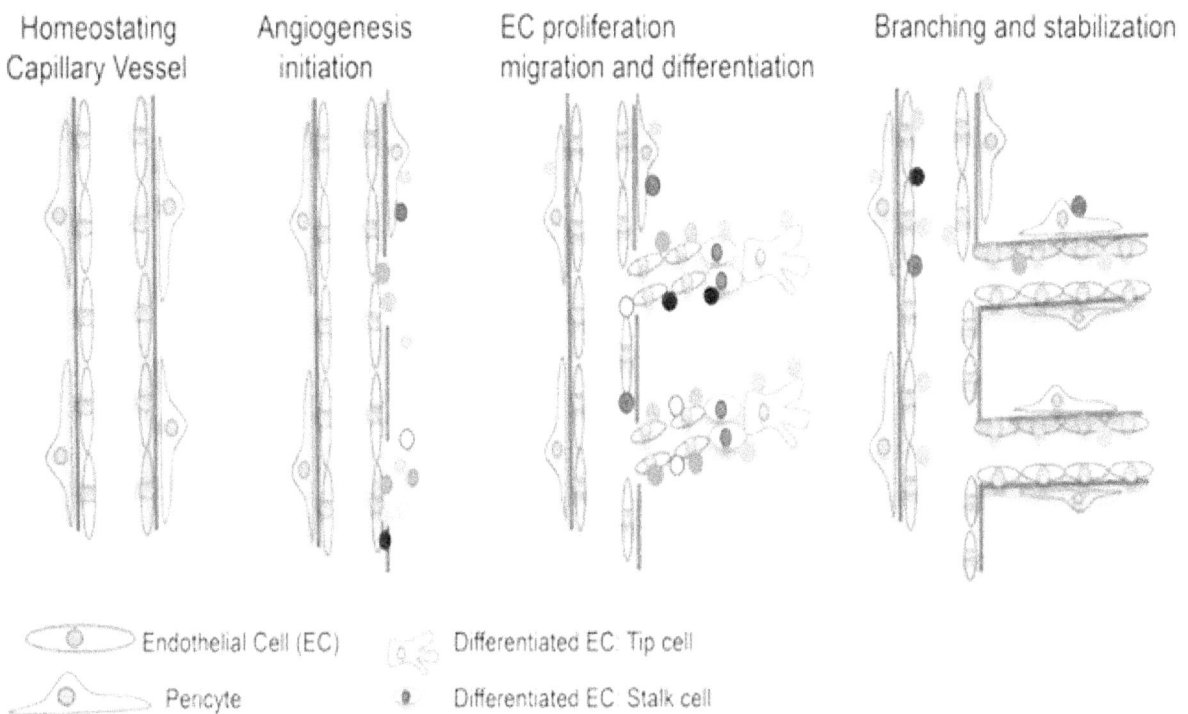

Fig. 2: Showing Role Different Growth Factors during Tissue regeneration

Source: Ehrenfest *et al.* (2009).

4

Clinical Implications of PRP

The PRP lead to tissue regeneration and stimulate the healing.

The various clinical implications are as following;

a. Cell Proliferation & Tissue Differentiation

- Promote Tenocyte & Tenocyte stem cells proliferation in vitro;
- Accelerate the proliferation rates of circulating stem cells such as bone marrow stem cells (BMSCs) and adipose derived stem cells (ADSCs) thereby accelerating tendon healing
- Positively influence cell attachment and spreading on the fibrin scaffold, as well as promoting cell proliferation
- TSCs differentiation into tenocytes.

b. Anabolic Effects

- Influence the metabolism of tendon cells,
- Increase total collagen synthesis in both tenocytes and TSCs
- specifically enhance the gene expression of collagen types I and III.
- Enhance the expression of COMP, decorin, and tenascin-C (tendon healing glycoproteins)
- Leukocytes in PRP may negatively affect the anabolic effects of PRP
- and may lead to scar formation by increasing the collagen type III/collagen type I ratio

c. Anti-Inflammatory Effects

- Induce the release of HGF, which is a major anti-inflammatory growth factor
- Increased VEGF and HGF expression in tendinopathy tendons
- Reduction in the levels of COX-1, COX-2, and PGE2,
    - o Pro-inflammatory cytokine,
    - o IL-6, and its ligand, CXCL-6, and IL-8
- Increase anti-inflammatory cytokine IL-10 &TGF-β levels.

d. Antibiotic Effects

- Active role in sepsis and fighting infection (including promoting the innate immune response).
- Significantly decreased bacterial growth, particularly of:
    - *MRSA,*
    - *P. acnes,*
    - *S. epidermidis*, and
    - *S. aureus.*

The PRP is Synergistic in combination and can be used with Stem cells & other tissue engineering modalities to enhance healing.

Basic science studies have consistently shown the beneficial effects of PRP including increased cell proliferation, increased expression of anabolic genes and proteins, and reduced inflammation.

The PRP promotes proliferative healing instead of inflammatory healing.

The clinical application of the Autologous PRP, is feasible because of

- Ease of Preparation
- No Ethical Issues
- Safety- Autologous
- Easily Accessible
- Low Cost- Affordability
- Ongoing Clinical Evidences:
    - Tendon Healing, Bone healing, Cartilage Healing, Wound healing, hair growth and many other cinical conditions.

5

Preparation of PRP

A. Basic Principles

The platelet separation is based upon Differential Centrifugation. The acceleration force is adjusted to sediment certain cellular constituents based on different specific gravity.

The Plasma mainly consist of RBC,WBC and Platelets. The RBC's have heaviest molecular weight and lightest being the WBC's. Hence a differential centrifugation will precipitate the RBC to the bottam of the tube and WBC to be the top layer beneath the plasma (Fig.3).

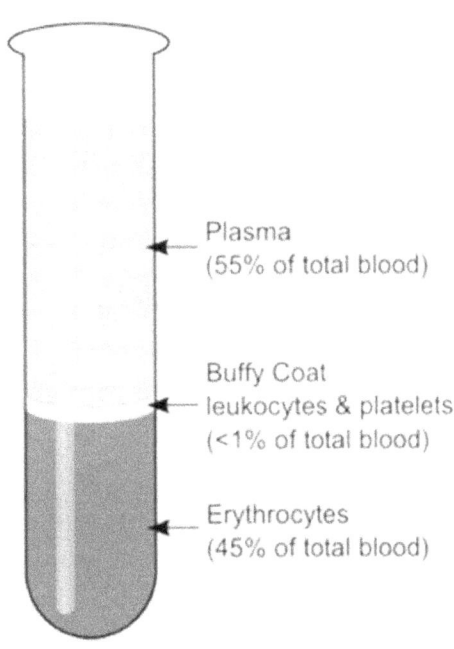

Plasma
(55% of total blood)

Buffy Coat
leukocytes & platelets
(<1% of total blood)

Erythrocytes
(45% of total blood)

**Figure 3: Showing Blood Fractionation:
Cells, whole blood, plasma.**

B. Methods for Preparation

It can be prepared by the two methods: PRP method or by the buffy-coat method

i. PRP Method:

A first spin is performed leading to separation of

- The Pure PRP (P-PRP) which is the Upper layer and superficial buffy coat, these are transferred to an empty sterile tube; and

- The second layer of Leucocyte rich PRP (L-PRP): The entire layer of buffy coat and few RBCs are transferred.

The second spin step is then performed.

'g' for second spin should be just adequate

: soft pellets (erythrocyte-platelet) is formed at the bottom of the tube.

The upper portion of the volume that is composed mostly of PPP (platelet-poor plasma) is removed.

Pellets are homogenized in lower 1/3rd (5 ml of plasma) to create the PRP (Platelet-Rich Plasma).

STEPS: Fig.4

1. Obtain WB by veni-puncture in acid citrate dextrose (ACD) tubes
2. Do not chill the blood at any time before or during platelet separation.
3. Centrifuge the blood using a 'soft' spin.
4. Transfer the supernatant plasma containing platelets into another sterile tube (without anticoagulant).
5. Centrifuge tube at a higher speed (a hard spin) to obtain a platelet concentrate.
6. The lower 1/3rd is PRP and upper 2/3rd is platelet-poor plasma (PPP). At the bottom of the tube, platelet pellets are formed.
7. Remove PPP and suspend the platelet pellets in a minimum quantity of plasma (2-4 mL) by gently shaking the tube

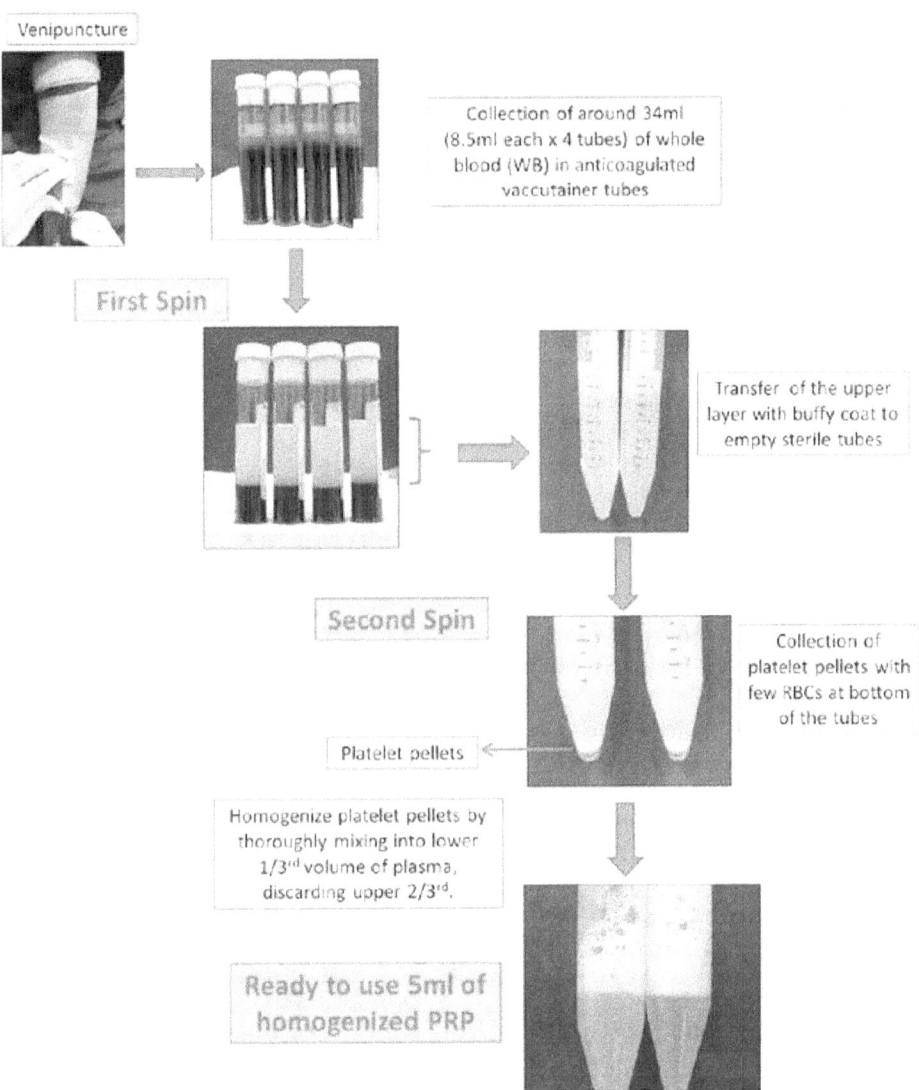

Figure 4: Showing PRP method.

ii. Buffy coat method,

Whole blood (WB) is centrifuged at a 'high speed' with subsequent collection of the buffy coat.

A buffy coat contains high concentration of leucocytes.

From small volume of WB (10 mL), a very thin layer of a buffy coat can be produced.

The difficulty lies in separating this thin buffy coat layer that contains mainly white blood cells (WBCs) and platelets, from the underlying RBC layer.

STEPS:

1. Whole Blood (WB) should be stored at 20°C to 24°C before centrifugation.
2. Centrifuge WB at a 'high' speed.
3. Three layers are formed because of its density:
   - Bottom layer consisting of RBCs,
   - Middle layer consisting of platelets and
   - WBCs and the top PPP layer.
4. Remove supernatant plasma from the top of the container.
5. Transfer the buffy-coat layer to another sterile tube.
6. Centrifuge at low speed to separate WBCs or use leucocyte filtration filter.

Anitua E in 1999 propagated the single spin method:

This consist of:

- 10-20ml WB from the patient.
- Addition of 10% tri-sodium citrate as anticoagulant
- Calcium chloride as activator
- RPM of 160g for 6 minutes.
- They achieved 2-3 fold increase in the Platelet concentration.

Pietrazzak WS and EppleyBL in 2005 propagated the double spin technique.

This consist of:

Collection of WB in anticoaugulant tube and

First spin is hard spin leading to separation of RBCs and Buffy coat

Second Spin is soft spin separating the PRP from PPP.

In 2009 FDA approved the Two stage PRP preparation methods, with

- Collection of the patient's whole blood (that is anticoagulated with citrate dextrose)
- Two stages of centrifugation, designed to separate the PRP aliquot from platelet-poor plasma and red blood cells.

Alissa et al (2010) Propagated the single stage centrifugation and used Thrombin as anticoagulant.

There is broad variability in the production of PRP by various concentrating equipment and techniques. In humans, the typical baseline blood platelet count is approximately 200,000 per μL; and the targeted therapeutic PRP concentrates should have the platelets by roughly five-fold.

There are commercial kits (Figure 5) available for the PRP and its subtype to be made.

There are also pre-programmed centrifuge machines (Figure 6) available to make these PRP.

Usually the Fresh autologous WB is collected (upto50ml) in these prefilled tubes and then centrifuged in the pre-programmed (with Pre-Set RPM and Time) manner. They are then activated by adding the calcium chloride and thrombin, to make a PRP gel.

Based on these, different authors have developed different methods by centrifuging at variable speeds for variable time. The table 3 shows the results in terms of Platelet count at the end of each method.

Study	Volume of WB (mL)	1st Centrifugation		2nd Centrifugation		Platelet count rise
		Force (RCF)	Time (min)	Force (RCF)	Time (min)	
Amable *et al.*	4.5	300	5	700	17	1.4×10^5 to 1.9×10^6 5.4-fold to 7.3-fold
Amanda *et al.*	3.5	100	10	400	10	$1.222 \pm 166 \times 10^3$ 5-fold
Khan *et al.*	478	3731	4	---	---	8.3×10^{10}
Stichter and Harker	250-450	1000	9	3000	20	80% Recovery
Landesberg *et al.*	5	200	10	200	10	5.57 to 9.35×10^5
Jo *et al.*	9	900	5	1500	15	$633.2 \pm 91.6 \times 10^3$ 4.2 times
Bausset	10	250	15	250	15	3.96 times
Tamimi *et al.*	8.5	160	10	400	10	630.2×10^3
Mazzocca *et al.*	27	1500 rpm	5	6300 rpm	20	472×10^3
Anitua *et al.*	4.5	460	8	Single spin only		2.67 times
Araki *et al.*	7.5	270	10	2300	10	189.6×10^4
Kececi *et al.*	9	250	10	750	10	679.9×10^3

RCF: Relative centrifugal force, WB: Whole blood

Table 3: Shows the Platelet count and achieved by different authors at variable centrifuge speeds and time.

Source:

Rachita Dhurat and MS Sukesh et al J Cutan Aesthet Surg. 2014 Oct-Dec; 7(4): 189–197.Principles and Methods of Preparation of Platelet-Rich Plasma: A Review and Author's Perspective.

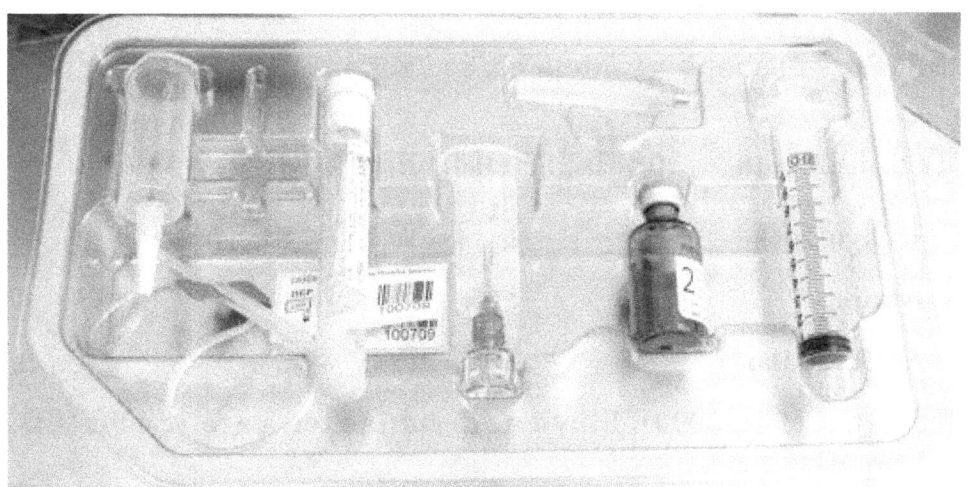

Figure 5: Showing a typical commercial kit for PRP Preparation

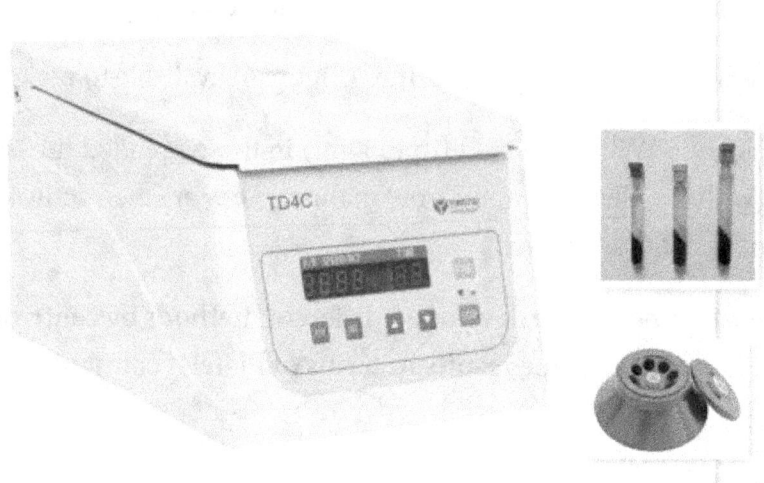

Figure 6: Showing a Pre- programmed centrifuge Machines.

The PRP devices can be usually divided into lower (2.5-3 times baseline concentration) and higher (5–9 times baseline concentration) systems.

The high-yielding devices include:

- Biomet GPS II and III (platelet count 3–8×);
- Harvest SmartPRep 2 APC + (4–6×);
- ArterioCyte-Medtronic Magellan (3–7×).

The lower concentration systems include:

- Arthrex ACP (2–3×),
- Cascade PPR therapy (1–1.5×),
- PRGF by Boitech Institute Vitoria, Spain (2–3×).
- Regen PRP (Regen Laboratory, Mollens, Switzerland)

C. There are two important issue in preparation of PRP

i. **Choice of Anticoagulant**

ii. **Choice of Activation**

    i. **Choice of Anticoagulant:**

       - **Landesberg R et al (2000): Ethylene di-amine tetra acetic acid (EDTA)**

It is more harmful than citrate in the preparation of PRP, based on the observation of large number of damaged platelets.

- **Marx RE (2001): Citrate dextrose-A is a preferable agent.**

  The citrate binds calcium and prevents coagulation whereas dextrose and other ingredients support platelet metabolism and viability.

- **Citrate phosphate dextrose is also useful for PRP preparation.**

ii. Choice of Activation:

Mechanism:

The activation causes the granules present in platelets to fuse to its cell membrane (**also called degranulation**).

Where the secretory proteins (e.g. PDGF, TGF-β etc.) are transformed to a bioactive state by the addition of histones and carbohydrate side chains.

The active proteins are then secreted, binding to transmembrane receptors of target cells, which include mesenchymal stem cells, osteoblasts, fibroblasts, endothelial cells and epidermal cells. These agonists bound transmembrane receptors then activate an intracellular signal protein that causes the expression of a gene sequence that directs cellular proliferation, matrix formation, osteoid production, collagen synthesis etc.

Thus provoking tissue repair and tissue regeneration

The active secretion of these growth factors by platelets begins within 10 min after activation, with more than 95% of the pre-synthesized growth factors secreted within 1 h

Agents:

They interact with leukocytes, endothelial cells and circulating bone marrow derived progenitor cells. The commonly used activation agents are:

- **10% calcium chloride and Thrombin**: an activator that allows polymerization of the fibrin into an insoluble gel which causes the platelets to degranulate and release indicated mediators and cytokines.

- **TRAP -Thrombin Receptor Activated Protein** (Regina Landsberg et al, 2005): It is a safe economic alternative to thrombin for preparation of PRP.

- **Bovine Thrombin:** Rick C. Tsay et al (2005) quantified the growth factors (PDGF and TGF β) released from PRP clotted with bovine thrombin

Self-Activation:

This concept is based on Autocrine and Paracrine self-activation processes.

This is based on:

- Regulated inflammatory Response
- Chemotaxis
- Athero-thrombosis
- Coagulation.

This promote the cellar differentiation, hence the regeneration.

Overall still there is no general consensus on the need for previous activation of platelets before

their application. Many authors use calcium or thrombin and some other apply platelets without being previously activated arguing the better results are obtained. We also propagate the use of self-activation, avoiding any risk of chemical damages.

D. Factors effecting PRP yield

i. **Draw of Blood**: The clotting process is influenced from the time of the draw.

   Preference is with a **Large Bore Needle**

   Downward trend in platelet counts with longer draw time*

   (Waters JH, Roberts KC. Database review of possible factors influencing point-of-care platelet gel manufacture. J Extra Corpor Technol. 2004;36:250–4)

ii. **Centrifuging: Faster separating techniques. Formula: g=(1.118x10-5) R S2 ; g is RCF, R radius of rotor in cm and S speed in RPM double spin - soft & hard.**

iii. **Temperature: Crucial for activation, Recommended: 21-24OC. Cooling retards platelet activation.**

(Macey M, Azam U, McCarthy D, Webb L, Chapman ES, Okrongly D, et al. Evaluation of the anticoagulants EDTA and citrate, theophylline, adenosine, and dipyridamole (CTAD) for assessing platelet activation on the ADVIA 120 hematology system. Clin Chem. 2002;48:891–9)

iv. **Anticoagulants**: Preserve platelets – functionality, integrity and morphology; platelet aggregation-pH & extracellular iCa concentration.

Sodium citrate Vs ACD-A - low (4.9) pH, High Citrate (24.4) ion/ml.

Citrate phosphate dextrose adenine (10% less effective than ACD-A)

EDTA - mostly avoided

(*Anitua E, Prado R, Sánchez M, Orive G. Platelet-rich-plasma: Preparation and formulation. Oper Tech Orthop. 2012;22:25–32.

**Callan MB, Shofer FS, Catalfamo JL. Effects of anticoagulant on pH, ionized calcium concentration, and agonist-induced platelet aggregation in canine platelet-rich plasma. American journal of veterinary research. 2009;70:472–7.

doi:10.2460/ajvr.70.4.472.)

v. **Activation:** This can be achieved through addition of Thrombin, calcium chloride or Mechanical trauma. Collagen is natural activator, and soft tissue usage will not need activation

(*Marlovits S, Mousavi M, Gabler C, Erdös J, Vécsei V, et al. A new simplified technique for producing platelet-rich plasma: A short technical note. Eur Spine J. 13:102–06)

vi. **Physiological factors:**

- **Age & Sex:** No effect (Weibrich G, Hansen T, Kleis W, Buch R, Hitzler WE. Effect of platelet concentration in platelet-rich plasma on peri-implant bone regeneration. Bone. 2004;34:665–71)

- **Haematocrit and Total platelet count: Influenced** (Woodell-May JE, Ridderman DN, Swift MJ, Higgins J. Producing accurate platelet counts for platelet rich plasma: Validation of a hematology analyzer and preparation techniques for counting. J Craniofac Surg. 2005;16:749–59)

A Standardized Preparation of PRP Can Be Achieved, Through Following

1. Draw blood in anticoagulant vacutainer tubes using BD Eclipse™ blood collection needle (Ref: 368607; BD Biosciences, India)

2. Set apart 1-2 mL for baseline cell counting including RBCs, platelets, WBCs and haematocrit.

3. Blood samples that are collected in ACD tubes should be inverted 5-10 times for proper mixing of the anticoagulant and blood. If the tube is not mixed, small fibrin clots may form, causing a falsely decreased platelet count.

4. *After 1st spin, measure the platelet count in RBCs and the supernatant to ensure optimal separation of platelets from the WB.

5. **If this does not happen, change the parameters like RPM and Time.

6. After first spin, if large volume of plasma is obtained, then it would need higher 'g' to concentrate platelets at the bottom of the tube (law of velocity).

7. After 2nd spin, measure the platelet count in PPP and PRP after adequately racking the tubes.

8. If higher concentration of platelets in platelet poor plasma (upper layer) or lower concentration in PRP (bottom layer) is observed, then the parameters are not optimal.

9. PRP must be separated from the PPP soon after centrifugation because the concentrated platelets will slowly diffuse into the PPP over time and would reduce the platelet count of the PRP preparation.

10. For counting the platelets in the final PRP concentrate, it must be re-suspended for at least 5-10 min to allow for equal distribution of platelets before counting.

11. To obtain a yield of platelet in PRP more than 10 lakhs/mL*

12. All variables like rpm, time and temperature should be standardized and consistency of platelet concentrate has to be maintained over the period at 900g x 5 mins for 1st centrifugation and 1000g x 10 mins for 2nd centrifugation at 16° C in a refrigerated centrifuge (eg: RemiCM8plus; Remiworld, India).

(* Rachita Dhurat and MS Sukesh, Principles and Methods of Preparation of Platelet-Rich Plasma: A Review and Author's Perspective J

6

Key Evidences for PRP

1970s: PRP was first developed.

1987: First used in Italy in an open heart surgery procedure.

1990s: PRP therapy began gaining popularity

The number of peer reviewed publications studying the PRP's efficacy has increased dramatically since **2007.**

2009: systematic review: Few randomized controlled trials that adequately evaluated the safety and efficacy of PRP treatments: concluded that PRP was "a promising, but not proven, treatment option for joint, tendon, ligament, and muscle injuries".[1]

2010: Cochrane analysis: use in sinus lifts during dental implant placement found no evidence that PRP offered any benefit.

2012: Cerza Am Journal Sports Med, level 1, randomized control trial concluded: Significantly better for OA knee than hyaluronic acid.

2013: More evidence was needed to determine PRP's effectiveness for hair regrowth.

2014: Cochrane analysis: use to treat musculoskeletal injuries found very weak (very low quality) evidence for a decrease in pain in the short term,

Up to three months and no difference in function in the short, medium or long term.

There was weak evidence that suggested that harm occurred at comparable, low rates in treated and untreated people.

2014: the *American Journal of Sports Medicine*: "Application of 3 consecutive PRP injections significantly improved symptoms and function in athletes with chronic patellar tendinopathy and allowed fast recovery and return to sport.

There was return to normal architecture of the tendon as assessed by MRI.

2015: meta-analysis PRP for osteoarthritic (OA) knee (551 studies): 9 worth considering:

Short term outcomes- PRP was not more efficacious than placebo (total WOMAC score) but was more efficacious than hyaluronic acid (HA) on that measure;

2016: systematic review and meta-analysis of randomized controlled clinical trials for PRP use to augment bone graft - only one study reporting a significant difference in bone augmentation, while four studies found no significant difference.

2016: results of basic science and preclinical trials have not yet been confirmed in large-scale randomized controlled trials.

Forogh B, Mianehsaz E, Shoaee S, Ahadi T, Raissi GR, Sajadi S. Effect of single injection of platelet-rich plasma in comparison with corticosteroid on knee osteoarthritis: a double-blind randomized clinical trial. The Journal of sports medicine and physical fitness. 2016;56(7-8):901.

The evidences now have gathered certainties over following issues related to PRP:

1. **Preparation**
2. **Site of deliveries**
3. **Relative Indication**
4. **Safety**

But still there are many uncertainties including:

1. **How Rich should be the PRP for therapeutic effects**
2. **Absolute indications for PRP therapy.**
3. **Dose as per the clinical diseases and disorders.**
4. **Exact Mechanism of the PRP.**
5. **Long term effects**

Chapter II

PRP for Wounds

1

Introduction

People tend to get injured and develop wound. Many times, these are associated with skin and underlying tissue loss. Without skin coverage, the underlying muscles, tendons and bones lay exposed and are at the huge risk of infection and necrosis. This may lead to their permanent loss. Many of them do not heal because of co-morbid conditions including old age, diseases such as diabetes; and neurogenic conditions. These wounds become a complex problem leading to non-healings and further morbidities. It is estimated that care of such wounds exceeds 50 billion dollars per year in US, which is 10 times of the WHO health care budget. The effective management of complex wounds presents a huge challenge for mankind. Throughout the world these wounds are managed with lots of variations & uncertainties. The treatment involve huge resources. Conventionally it includes surgical interventions, intense local care and medical treatments. More so they may need skin gratings and reconstructions. Newer pursuits to manage these wounds have led to creation of more complex treatments These treatments can only be imparted at Higher health care centers by highly trained experts such as plastic surgeons. These procedures are associated with donor site morbidities and risk of anesthesia and operation. Many a times with active infections, uncontrolled blood sugar and in children it may not be possible to undertake such procedures. The reconstructed skins do not have the same texture and strength as natural skin specially in areas such as sole, and are associated problem of recurrence. There is still no common solution which is effective in dealing with predictable outcome, in such complicated situations and can be imparted uniformly by all doctors with little training and resources.

The regenerative medicine offers a ray of hope. Attempts are witnessed since last two decades to identify the properties of Platelet and platelet rich plasma in the wound healing. The PRP has excellent regenerative property and initiates wound repair by releasing locally acting growth factors via α-granules degranulation.

2
Rationale

The tissue repair starts with clot formation and platelet degranulation, leading to the release of the growth factors (GFs). The alpha granules in turn liberates the growth factors responsible for biological properties of PRP towards wound healing. This cascade enhances tissue repair mechanisms such as chemotaxis, cell proliferation, angiogenesis, extracellular matrix deposition, and remodeling. The secretory proteins contained in the α-granules of platelets include platelet-derived growth factor (PDGF-AA, BB, and AB isomers), transforming growth factor-β (TGF-β), platelet factor 4 (PF4), interleukin-1 (IL-1), platelet-derived angiogenesis factor (PDAF), vascular endothelial growth factor (VEGF), epidermal growth factor (EGF), platelet-derived endothelial growth factor (PDEGF), epithelial cell growth factor (ECGF), insulin-like growth factor (IGF) [osteocalcin (Oc), osteonectin (On), fibrinogen (Ff), vitronectin (Vn), fibronectin (Fn), and thrombospondin-1 (TSP-1). These growth factors aid healing by triggering cell a chain of cellular signalling and molecular response leading to angiogenesis. In addition, the macrophages too are attracted to the site and built on the lost host defense. Many studies have also demonstrated antimicrobial activity, including against Escherichia coli, Staphylococcus aureus, including methicillin-resistant Staphylococcus aureus, Candida albicans, and Cryptococcus neoformans.

3

Key Evidences

Pre-clinical studies in mice and rabbits have been reported which indicates safety and efficacy of PRP use in chronic ulcers and wounds.

Many clinical studies have been reported in last decade, on utilization of PRP for wound healing.

The PRP is being used mostly as a local application either as gel or liquid or spray. These are externally activated and is used as an adjunct to the conventional therapy for wound management, mostly as local dressings. Only 4 studies in last decade used PRP in other form as local sub-cutaneous injections. Tzeng et al used it as a spray.

All of them have used PRP as adjunct to therapies including along with vacuum sealants or followed by immediate skin gratings as by Tzeng et al and Sano et al. The local gel application has found to have ease and inexpensive by Ramos et al. PRP have been used for different tyes of wounds like chronic non-healing wounds, chronic venous ulcers, diabetic ulcers, pressure ulcers, burn wounds, compound fractures or even a post malignancy wound. The results for most of the study are favorable and hints at superior outcome. Systematic reviews by Martinez in 2009 & 2012, Villela in 2010 have been done. In addition, meta-analysis has also been conducted on PRP and its role on wound healing for different types of wounds by Marissa in 2011, Cobos in 2013 and Wang in 2014. The studies included have used PRP gel as local applications. The results are variable from equivocal to superior benefits. The initial ones conducted in 2009 reported the role of PRP to be inconclusive. But as more evidence kept on building, the recent ones indicate a positive role of PRP by shortening the wound healing duration, hospital stay and control of pain and to some extent infection too. They have concluded about the safety and efficacy of PRP. No major risks have been identified. Variations exists as per the Preparation of PRP, Form of PRP and even the use of other modalities along with PRP.

These studies are indicating that PRP led therapy has the potential for an ideal treatment.

Few critical gaps still exit, there is no single most efficient preparation method is identified till now. Similarly imparting the PRP therapy has lots of variations in terms of the dose, duration and end point.

4

Our Experience

There is a strong need for development and evoking therapy which is single, simple, cheaper and effective in such conditions without involving the surgical procedures and drugs. Wide application of such product is only possible if it has ease of preparation, safety and wide reproducibility. The fresh autologous PRP has all the potentials to be an ideal product for wound healing. Till now the PRP have been used clinically in wounds, more as a local application than as a definite regenerative medicine product.

We undertook a project on developing Autologous PRP as a monotherapy for Wound care, independent of major surgeries, Drugs and intense local dressing. Since 2009 we had been involved with different aspects of development of PRP therapy. We intended to keep t as simple as possible so that it can be done with ease and have a huge access for reproducibility, even in the hands of minimally trained health workers.

Finally, in 2014 we evolved a protocol for PRP therapy, incorporating easy Preparation method, standardized dose, schedules, delivery and safety. This is later copyrighted by the name of **"Sandeep's Technique for Assisted Regeneration of Skin"** (STARS) therapy. It has been developed with an intention of single uniform solution for all wounds. It is a very low cost, effective and efficient therapy for treatment of even complex wounds, where even the hope for salvages are lost. The Product used is autologous PRP, made from Patients own fresh low volume venous blood. Hence in a way, the Patient themselves are healers for their own misery. Almost an ideal solution for one of most complex human health problem has been developed!.

Subsequent Chapter explains the details of STARS therapy.

Chapter III
ATLAS of STARS Therapy

1

Introduction

Aim

To develop an Ideal solution for wound management

Objectives

A wound therapy which is:

- **SAFE:**
  - o No additional risks of Drugs/Surgery.
  - o Can be given safely to Persons with severe co-morbidities such
  - o Diabetes, Ischemic Heart diseases, Renal Failures etc.
  - o Use autologous body product with no risk of transmitted diseases.
  - o Minimally Invasive procedure.
- **EFFECTIVE:**
  - o Highly predictable results for all/most of the wounds
  - o Is able to tackle complications including infection.
  - o Can take up the current solutions to next level like regeneration in gangrenous or near gangrenous tissues.
- **EFFICIENT:**
  - o Low cost & low on Resource consumptions.
  - o Easy accessibility: Only Autologous, PRP with no additives.
  - o No/minimal hospitalizations.

- **EASILY REPRODUCIBLE:**
  - o Can be imparted by all health care providers -Physician/Nurse/Paramedic etc.
  - o Low cost technology accessible to all the level of health care - from Primary to Territory.
  - o Involves Simple Technique.
  - o Can be done on Outdoor/Day care basis.

Choice of Regenerative Medicine Product as Ideal Solution

The best chance for tissue repair, regeneration and revivals is with the Regenerative Medicine.

It is assisting the normal regenerative process.

As mentioned earlier, the 3 most common regenerative medicine products (currently in vogue)

- Stem cells – Embryogenic, Adult or Bioengineered
- Mesenchymal stem cells, and
- PLATELETS

Out of these Platelets are most easily accessible. It is a very cost-effective preparation as compared to others and can be prepared with low volume of venous blood.

The PRP preparation does not need any cell cultures, hence no sophisticated laboratories are required. There are no controversies to its use including any ethical issues and approvals

The PRP form has been now widely used clinically for regeneration of many tissues in various disorders such Fracture impairment, Tendinopathies etc.

The PRP in form of gels are commercially available too, approved for wound management.

Platelets have alpha granules which are rich source of many Cytokines and Growth factors.

These include EGF epidermal growth factor, FGF fibrocyte growth Factor, VEGF vascular endothelium growth factor, TGF transforming Growth Factor, PDGF platelet derived growth factors. It has IL4; IL6 cytokines too.

There are 2 key roles of platelets, after injury—initially it triggers the cascade mechanism for clot formation and -subsequently takes part in inflammation and these growth factors as listed above triggers the repair & regeneration process. This induces Angiogenesis, over which the Fibrocytic and Collagen cells form the collagen tissue, and fill up the defect. This Inflammatory process led by PRP induced healing is IL4, hence is said to be predominantly Collagen led.

The Platelets through its growth factors and cytokines acts by Cellular signaling and Molecular responses and do not have nucleus so it has no potentials for inducing abnormal cell divisions and hence any cancers.

The principle of wound healing is a reparative process initially the wound defects are filled up with granulation tissue and the natural epithelization starts from margin.

The STARS therapy is based on hypothesis that regenerative assistance through PRP, can be created for both the above as following:

1. The inflammatory pathways in the presence of the PRP liberated cytokines, in initial phase should stimulate the Proliferative inflammation leading the angiogenesis, and granulation formation. Hence speeding the filling up of the defects. It should also induces the inflammations in non-healing wounds, where the process of repair has ceased.
2. The regeneration of the neo-epithelization (skin) assisted by PRP infiltration is through liberation of growth factors particularly the endodermal and epidermal. It also leads fibro-collagen based tissue formations, then a pure fibrotic or cicatrized tissue (scars), which is more useful and natural.

Hence PPR led STARS therapy should be an Ideal solution for Wounds.

2

The Technique

Step 1

Selection of Case

Inclusion: All Wounds including Acute post traumatic, Compound fractures, Burst abdomen, Post-operative, Diabetic ulcer, Bed sore, Venous ulcers, Non-healing Ulcers. Wounds associated with infections and/or developing gangrenous/necrotic changes etc

Exclusions:

- Any Bleeding Disorder
- Any Haematological Oncology.
- Haemoglobin less than 10gm%*
- Platelet count- sub normal (less than 1 lac/cu mm)
- Anyone who is unfit for repeated collection of blood, for any reasons.

Wound Exclusion: Associated with Local Malignancy such as squamous cell carcinoma etc.

Caution

* if the Hb% is less than 10 gm% than it is built up by suitable treatment to 10gm% or more, before the start of STARS therapy.

Step 2

Collection of blood

20 ml of venous blood is withdrawn under all aseptic precautions

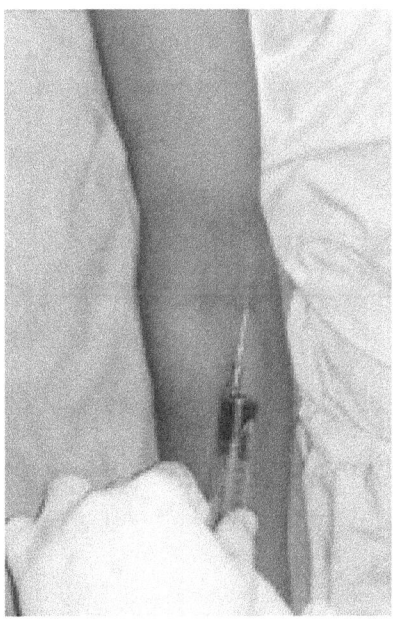

Figure 7: Showing Blood being withdrawn from antecubital vein

Step 3

Transfer of Blood:

Transfer into 4/8 tubes/bulbs (single EDTA/Citrate).

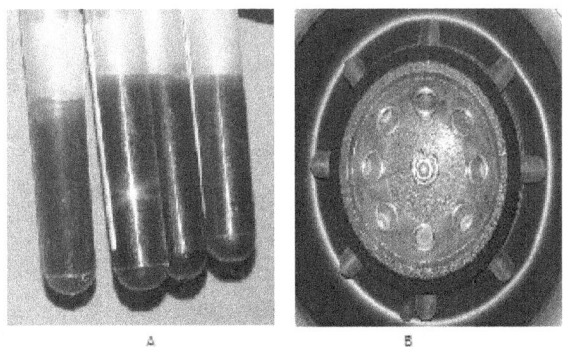

Figure 8: A. Showing transfer of equal quantity of blood in 4 bulbs &
B. Placement in the centrifuge machine loading with counter balancing

Step 4

Centrifuge -1

A. First Spin: 1200 RPM x 10 minutes.

B. Transfer & Collect upper Buffy layer in another tube.

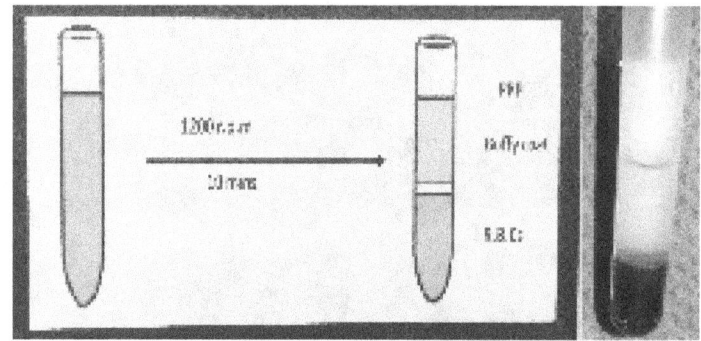

Figure 9: Showing separation of blood into Buffy coat and RBC layer

Step 5

Centrifuge – 2

A. Second Spin: 2000 RPM x 10 minutes.

B. The upper half is carefully aspirated with a syringe and the lower clear fluid is PRP with platelet pellet is homogenously gently mixed & then aspirated into a 5ml syringe.

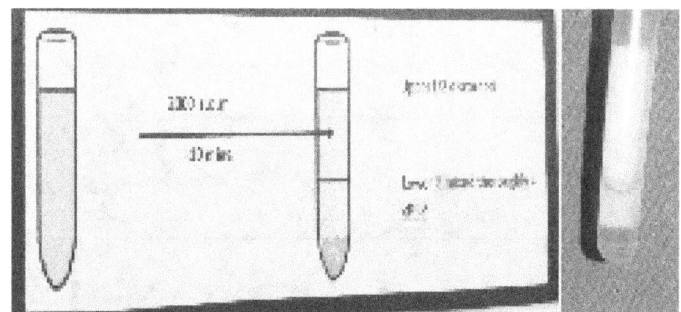

Figure 10: Showing Further separation into u ½ of mainly WBC and Lower PRP

Step 6

A. Wound Preparation.

- Clean the wound with normal saline.

- Clean the surrounding skin/margin up to 1cm wit Povidone iodine 2% or similar antimicrobial solution. (Figure A)

- Normal saline & apply 70% alcohol (eg: Spirit/Sterlium) and let it dry. (Figure B)

- Do not remove any tissue including dead & necrotising or peel off the newly forming delicate skin.

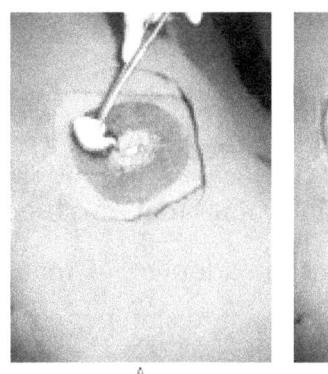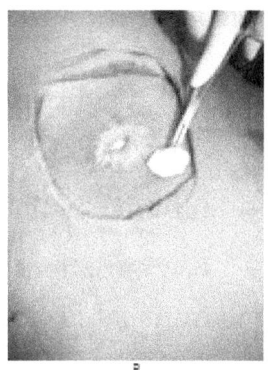

Figure: 11 A. Margin Preparation with Povidone Iodine.

B. Further cleaning with Alcohol and normal saline.

B. For Infected Wounds

Take a Pus swab for culture & sensitivity, after removal of dressing (on weekly basis)

Do not perform any debridement's; any slough etc naturally coming off can be gently removed by picking it up with forceps.

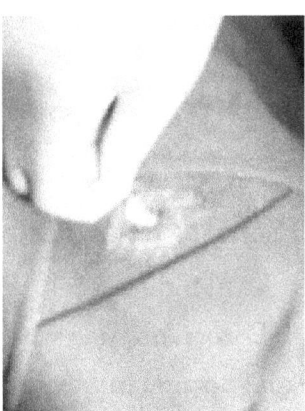

Figure 12: Showing Swab Collection for Culture & Sensitivity

CAUTION

Do not attempt to physically peel the scab.

If need be to remove the overlying scab: soak with Chlorhexadine gluconate & Cetrimide solution such as Savlon and let be gently lifted off.

Step 7

Local Infiltration with PRP

- Transfer all the PRP into a 2/5 ml disposable Syringe.

- Attach a 22G/24G needle.

- Infiltrate in the wound margin as shown in the Figure A.

- Few variations are adopted, as many a times Patients feel severe pain if penetration is done from hard skin, so hard skin penetration should be avoided to reach the regenerating margins. These could be from the wound side (Figure D) or from normal skin (Figure C)

- Infiltrate 0.2ml per 1 cm of length.

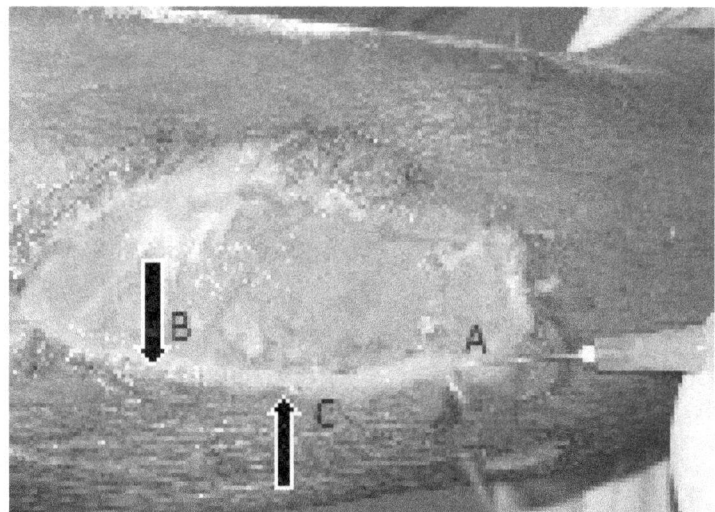

Figure: 13 Showing way to infiltrate PRP

A: Side ways

B. Direct into neo skin

C. From normal into neo-skin

CAUTION

- Ensure there is no leakage of fluid.
- Ensure there is no dehiscence of wound margin epithelizing skin.

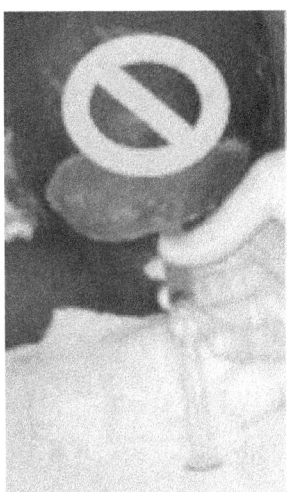

Figure 14: Do not infiltrate in wound

Step 8

Progressive Infiltrations

- Progressive infiltrations are done, in the healing wound margins; as shown in figure on every 4th day, using same technique as before in step 7

- END POINT: When the wound is healed completely or is small enough, usually less than 1 square cm to heal spontaneously.

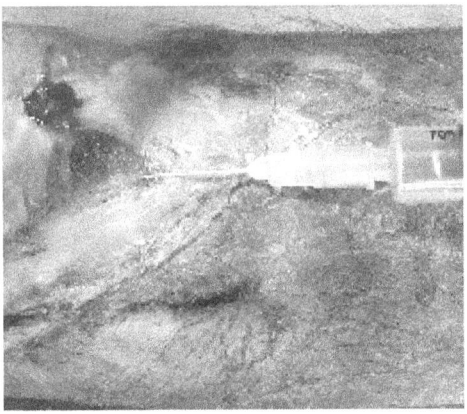

Figure: 15 Showing Infiltrations into the progressive regenerating skin margins

---

CAUTION

An earlier end point lead to residual Cicatrized healing.

Stars – Therapy

Summary of Technique

- **Blood Sample:** 20 ml Autologous Venous blood
- **Preparation into PRP:** Double spin centrifuge method
- **Form**: Fresh prepared Liquid form
- **Delivery:** Local Infiltration in regenerating skin Margin:
  o Subcutaneous Injection by 22G 10ml Syringe/Insulin Syringe.
- **Dose**: Progressive wound margin at a distance of 1 cm
  - 0.2 to 0.5 ml/1 cm every 4th day.
- **End point:** Till wound healed/less than 1 sq. cm

3

The Clinical Protocols

A. Local Dressings

a. Occlusive Dressing is done. after covering the wound with moist normal saline gauges.

b. The Dressing are changed daily or on alternate days, depending on the soakage's and discharges from the wound.

CAUTION

No Antimicrobial or any other solution is used locally over the wounds.

If the wounds are dirty (due to road side accidents etc), they are given daily immersion for 1/2 hr in a diluted solution of warm water and chlorhexidine Gluconate and Cetrimide, subsequently rinsed with normal saline and dressed with normal saline dressings.

B. Drugs

a. Only tablets of vitamin C are given to be chewed 6-8 hourly/day.

b. All other drugs as required for management of co-morbidities are routinely given as per prescriptions.

CAUTION

Use of Antibiotics:

- Routinely no antibiotics are given even for infected wounds.

- In infected wounds Pus Culture & Sensitivity tests are done weekly; till it become negative, and if at any time the wound deteriorates than antibiotics are started.

Use of Analgesics:

- A Visual Analogue scoring (VAS) on a scale of 10 is done for pain.

- If the pain is more than 7 only than I/V analgesics are prescribed.

- If pain is in the range of 3–7 than oral analgesics are prescribed on SOS basis.

C. Choice for Surgical Interventions

- No debridement's are done, gentle removal of loose slough or necrotic tissue is preferred.

- If the dry gangrene is established than only removal of that part is done.

- Whenever the wounds are found suitable for Plastic surgical options like skin grafting or flap coverages; an option of surgical reconstruction is offered to the Patient, and

  o   if he wants to undergo surgery the STARS therapy is discontinued and surgery undertaken.

  o   The surgical reconstruction can be augmented with PRP infusion at the bed of wound and at the suture sites.

Summary for Clinical Protocols

- No Complicated Dressings: SALINE Moist dressings- daily/alt days.

- For unclean wounds: Savlon soaks/Bath.

- No Regular Antibiotics:

  Repeated Cultures - every week.

  Start Antibiotics - If life threatening, Co-morbidities or

  Worsening of wound infection.

- No Regular Analgesics/anti-inflammatory: SOS only

- No Surgical Debridement: Preservation of every bit,

- No Surgical Reconstruction: Option given for surgical reconstruction

Only

- **Tablets of Vitamin C: 1x 3-4 times/day (to be chewed).**

- **PRP infiltrations on every 4th day.**

After Care

At end of treatment some after care is also needed.

These include:

- There is tendency for healed skin to be dry and itchy.

- This can be prevented by gentle application of petroleum jelly creams over the dry skin regularly over the skin

- Formation of a thick residual scab/keratinization's. Avoid intense peeling or surgically removal of these residual scabs which may be hard, and with these actions there is risk of underneath newly formed skin to get peeled off. We allow patients to use soap or place a gauze piece soaked in Cetrimide/Chlorhexidine combination solution (Savlon) over the scab for 15-30 minutes, and once the scab becomes soft; it can be gently lifted away. If a raw surface emerges a saline soaked occlusive dressing can be done.

- The immature skin takes about 3–6 weeks to completely mature further. Till such time it should be protected with soft coverings. Some discoloration remains, probably due to collagen tissue the skin appears lighter. This may take months to normalize.

- Usually no spontaneous wound dehiscence has been observed in a well healed wound through STARS therapy, including in the Soles, even after full weight bearing. This due to a better skin quality than the grafted ones. Though it is advisable to protect such skins from any further damages/injuries' particularly in diabetes.

- The skin formed had full sensations, even in tropical ulcers which healed almost every patient reported return of some sensation. This recovery could be speculated to regeneration of some neural tissues as well.

4

Development & Rationale

Limitation of Current Trends

The current evidences mostly use PRP as local dressing, adjunct to standard wound care management inclusive of drugs and surgeries.

Despite the clinical application gaining, there is lack of Standardization, particularly in terms of:

- PRODUCT: PRP – Fresh/Frozen-thawed; LR - PRP ; PPP etc.
- PREPARATION:
  - o Variable methods are used for preparation leading to a concentration unto 3 to 10 times.
  - o Induction of Activation or Self-Activation – Clinical utility not clear.
- FORM: Different forms are being used such as
  - o Activated GEL/LIQUID/SPRAY
- Delivery:
  - o Mostly as LOCAL APPLICATION over the wound.
- DOSE:
  - o Qquantity – UNCERTAIN
  - o Repeat dose: Variable: From once to 7th day to 3 monthly.
- END POINT:
  - o VARIED, No certain definite end point.

The Game Changer

PRP as Mono-therapy and mainstay management for wounds

Overview:

- Product: Autologue PRP.
- Preparation:
    - From: 20 ml venous blood-
    - Double spin Method
    - Form: Fresh prepared Liquid
- Delivery:
    - Local infiltration through 22/24 G needle.
- Technique:
    - Subcutaneous in the progressively healing margin at a distance of 1 cm
- Dose:
    - 0.2 to 0.5 ml/1 cm
        - to be repeated on 4th day.
- End point:
    - Till wound healed/or less than 1 sq. cm

STARS therapy development involves standardization as above based on certain Rationale and Results of continuous piloting over last decade.

The whole rationale for development was focused on meeting the aims and objective towards quest for ideal wound management solution.

1. The Product – Autologous PRP

The regenerative medicine product used in stars therapy is the Fresh Autologous PRP.

This is chosen for the facts that:

- It is absolutely safe there is no issue of any transmission of disease, as its autologous in nature.
- For the same reason, there is no need for testing of drawn blood too.
- Being autologous in nature there is no issue of accessibility & availability. It is available with the Patient itself.

- As the freshly prepared liquid form is used, hence there is no issue of it to be activated by adding certain additives and enzymes, which makes it easy to be use product.

- As it is made from the Patient own blood, the cost involved is just towards preparation and is very low, unlike commercial PRP products.

2. Method of PRP Preparation

A. Low volume blood:

Only 20 ml of venous blood is used for preparation of PRP in STARS therapy, unlike many others who use up to 50 ml. This yields about 2-4 ml of PRP which is mostly sufficient to cover a moderate wound up to 20–25 sq.cms.

The low volume is withdrawn, as the procedure is repeated frequently almost twice a week, so there should not be any effect on Patient due to repeated blood withdrawals, particularly the psychological.

In very exceptional circumstances when wounds are very large high volume up to 50 ml is taken.

B. Double spin method:

A very basic FDA approved method of double spin is used to prepare the PRP.

This with intentions to keep to the minimal specifications and resource. A simple machine which can accommodate 4 or 8 tubes with maximum RPM of about 2000–3000, is sufficient.

The quality of PRP is dependent on the concentrate of platelet. There is no clarity in the literature about exact Platelet concentrate in the plasma to qualify as Platelet Rich Plasma. A Strength anywhere between 3 to 10 times have been said to be enough to level the plasma as Platelet Rich Plasma.

The PRP Samples prepared in the STARS therapy are randomly tested and the Platelet concentrate in it had been found to be 3-8 times of normal values.

This Platelet count in PRP is independent of the previous blood values of Patient.

Hence the concentrate achieved by the double spin centrifuge method as used for PRP generation, meets the criteria of PRP.

All the PRP prepared are pure PRP with no leucocyte richness

As the double centrifuge method is simplest one, to prepare PRP and easily reproducible, requiring just a low RPM centrifuge machine, we have adopted it in the STARS technique.

3. The Dose of PRP

The total dose of PRP is between 2-4ml of PRP, in each session.

The key limitation is as the PRP is prepared from only 20ml of venous blood in each session, hence the total PRP available is about 2ml to 4ml.

This 2ml -4 ml is infiltrated as 0.2ml to 0.5 ml, at a distance of minimum 1 cm, though in large wounds this may get more spread up to a distance of 1.5-2cm.

In the growing neo-epithelization in which PRP is infiltrated the fluid should hold. The dose of 0.2ml is limited by this fact.

Few Problems are commonly noticed during infiltration:

- Leakage of PRP fluid:
  o To avoid this a only very small amount of PRP should be infiltrated.
  o Similarly, very small gauge needle (22/24G) is used to minimize the leaks and keep pain of infiltration to minimum. We have recently shifted to insulin syringes for the purpose of infiltration now.
  o PRP infiltrations can be more proximal in very precarious/fragile neo- skin regenerating margins.
- Pain during infiltration: Few Patients feel intense pain, particularly in first few infiltrations. This is seen mainly in Patients with chronic wounds with severe fibrosis at margins. These margins do not have space to expand and infusion of fluid and fluid infiltration leads to severe stretch pain.

  To avoid this, we have used local anesthetic creams, but with limited success. Better solutions are:

  o Choose appropriate approach out of the 3 ways as shown in technique section (Figure Number 13) for infiltrating the PRP into margins. The choice should from the area which are soft, so that the needle penetration is almost effortless and pain free. Ultimate aim is to infuse PRP in neo epithelizing tissue.
  o Initially just infiltrate a drop and let the tissue expand, later appropriate amounts up to 2ml can be infiltrated.
- In cases where the wound is very large we do different sessions at different sites, but usually do not exceed the above dosage, in each sitting.
- Similarly, in cases of multiple wounds; different days/alternate days may be selected for each wound treatment in the beginning.

4. Scheduling & Repeat/Follow up Dose

The PRP is repeated every 4th day in the STARS therapy.

In the literature, the repeat dose of PRP is not standardized till now and is varying from stat dose to be repeated on 7th day; to even repeated after 21 days or more.

The logic for these repeat dose is that the life of platelets is about 8–10 days, so 7–8 days should be able to sustain the active platelets at the site. But this contrary to the fact that the activation process of Platelets involves its destruction facilitating the liberation of alpha granules immediately after activation. Hence the life of Platelet cannot be the basis of repeat dose.

In our therapy, the "follow up/repeat doses" is based on two evidences:

- The PRP is targeted to stimulate the Proliferative healing. Hence the best time would be when the proliferative stage of wound healing, peaks. As per evidences in the literature this is 4th day (Figure 16 A). This is the time when angiogenesis and neo-epithelization triggers, hence it should repeatedly be stimulated towards regeneration, which van be achieved by the GF's from PRP.

- In our study on tendon healing assisted by PRP in Rabbit model, the inflammatory load estimation by the values of C-Reactive Proteins on different days from 1 to 21, were analyzed. We found the inflammation peaks on 3rd day and after that it tends to plateau to for 4-7 days and then is normal after 21 days. (Figure 16 B). This also prompted us to have a repeat/follow up dose of PRP on 4th day with the intention to trigger proliferative phase, specially for inducing healing in chronic non-healing wounds.

- We initially adopted 7th day protocol but results were not as per our desires, so after meticulous working, we figured that perhaps the 4th day would be the better choice and start repeat doses on 4th day. The results of STARS therapy improved significantly, once this was adopted as a protocol.

- In few cases, where wound defects were filled up and superficial epithelization was remaining, we deviate from the 4th day repeat protocol to 7th day protocol.

  Mostly this was done for outdoor care facilitation. A difference in wound healing rate and quality was noted. It not only slowed down but risk of infection also increased.

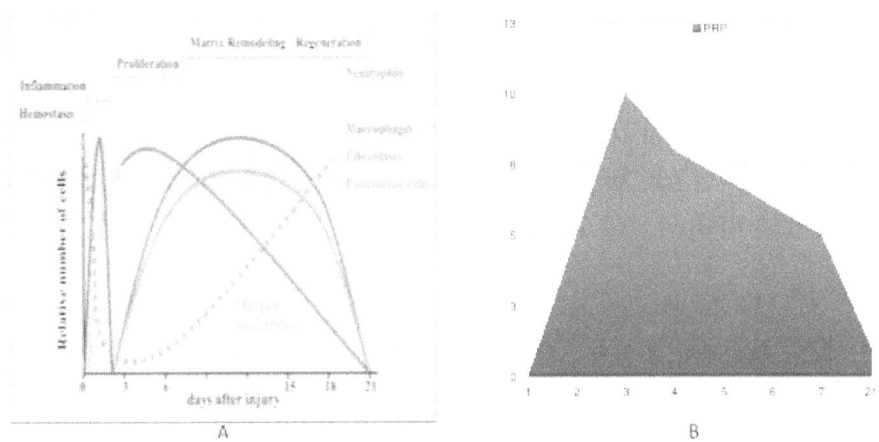

Figure 16: A. Showing Peaking of Proliferative Phase on day 4ᵗʰ, during wound healing.

B. Showing correlation between CRP – value and days.

5. The Delivery

Local (Subcutaneous) Infiltration.

The method of delivery of PRP in STARS technique is the most innovative step incorporated.

The most common method of delivery used currently is in the form of local gel application.

PRP being a blood product, we had a doubt regarding if it can control or promote infection. We conducted a microbiological laboratory test in which we used PRP as a culture media and found that bacteria tend to grow in concentrations as shown in Figure 17.

Based on this we conclude that local application of it could be risk factor for local infection.

Prompted by this key finding we also looked into the presence of any bacteria in the PRP prepared by us. The reports were negative, convincing us that PRP liquid is aseptic perse.

Not venturing to take any further risk for infection by using the liquid PRP locally, decided to infiltrate them deep into the wounds at equidistance. Though got results which were encouraging but not good enough also majority of liquid would just flow out of the wound immediately.

Based on these findings, also on the evidence of PRP liquid form being used for Orthobiologics and the platelet properties, we built another hypothesis that as the Platelets have so many growth factors including the angiogenetic, endodermal and epithethelial growth factor, perhaps it has a huge potential as a regenerative product than more of a repair product.

Its application on/in the wounds may not be the right manner to use PRP towards its regenerative potentials.

The better way would be to use it to assist the regenerating skin, and that would in turn cover the wound gradually, at the same time the cytokines would take care of good inflammation leading to healthy granulation formations.

Hence, we shifted to the site of infiltration to periphery of the wound in the margins. And as the margins grew inwards we also kept on infiltrating the progressively growing wound margin.

This was the major shift in the usage of PRP in wounds, and it proved to be spot on, as very soon the results yield a hugely better outcomes.

The subcutaneous infiltration in the wound margin lead to a typical pattern of wound healing induced by PRP, which is discussed further in the section of Pathology of STARS led wound healing.

Additionally, this form of injection is known to almost all the health care providers and with very little help they were able to do the same very easily, making the whole procedure easily reproducible in their hands.

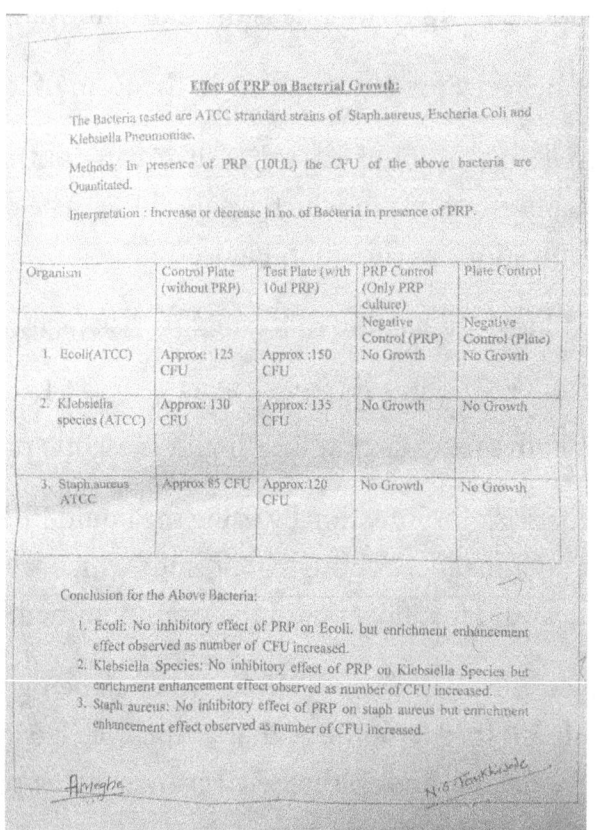

Figure 17: Showing the Report bacterial cultures in PRP and bacterial growths in it.

6. The End Point for STARS Therapy

The end point in the STARS therapy is when the wound is completely healed or the wound is small enough (less than 1 square cm) to be left for spontaneous healing without the risk of fibrosis and contractures.

We have noted few not so desirable outcomes if this end points are varied in terms of delays, missing doses or early end point. These are:

- Wound healing getting delayed,

- Mild infection reappearing and

- Wound healing with cicterization and secondary scars. (Figure 18A, B, C, D)

Hence it is advisable that the end point should be achievement of complete healing with full coverage of wound with epithelized tissue.

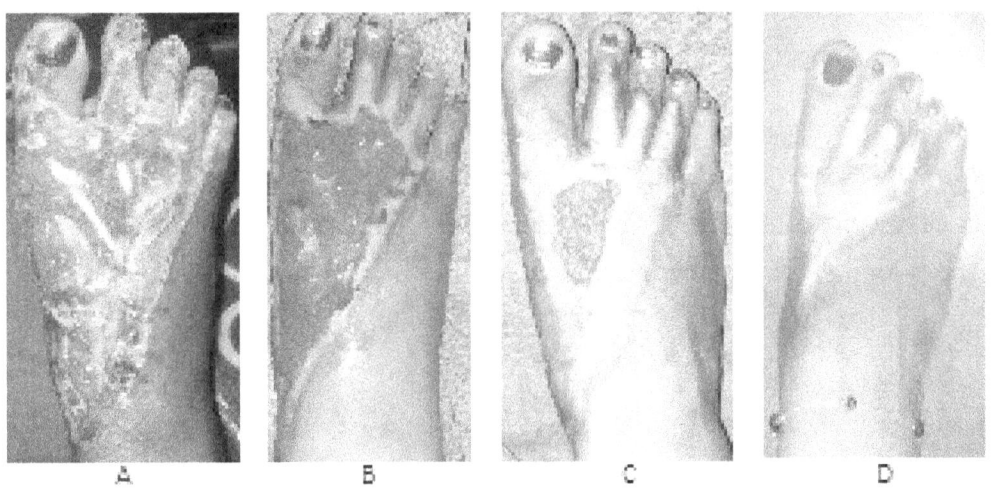

Figure 18: A: After foot injury.
B: Showing good progressive healing.
C: Patient abandoned the treatment at this point- Good skin regeneration is seen
D: On complete healing: Residual Scarring due to fibrosis formation is seen.

7. Moist Saline Occlusive Dressing

The STARS therapy, Propagates and uses no intense dressings with anti-microbial agents etc. It uses only moist saline coverage over wounds and keep it occlusive with firm compression bandaging.

It is essential to keep the wounds moist for them to survive and heal. We advocate the same and have used only moist saline dressing to cover the wound. The reasons are:

- Creation & preservation of a conducive natural environment, as triggered and induced by PRP, including the biochemical milieu. The saline being near normal fluid with neutral pH helps to maintain this. Moist saline is near isotonic aseptic solution, and if at all; it will have a minimal external influence on the wound, hence allowing the PRP induced changes to dominate/persist during the healing of wound.

- As the infiltration of PRP is made in the wound margin and growth factors are released, they tend to bring in the changes in/to the wound, particularly the precarious granulation tissue and neo-epithelization. The dryness and subsequent removal of dressings will damage both. The moist saline coverage with gentle compression protects them

- The dressings with antimicrobial agents or other chemical/ionic agents, changes the local environments including the pH, which may be not conducive for the growth factors to act.

  A change in local environment by external biological or chemical application interfere with building of such natural conducive environments.

These dressing are changed preferably on alternate days, but if they are soaked or foul smelling than they may need daily or on as need, changes.

8. Vitamin C

The main intention of including Tablet of Vitamin C in STARS therapy protocol is to give a feeling of satisfaction to the patients, that they are taking some medicine, sort of Placebo effect.

Vitamin C is chosen because:

- It Is one of the safest Vitamin which can be given.
- The Oral Preparation of it can be sucked or chewed.
- These preparations are of very palatable, so acceptable to everyone.
- Vitamin C aids in Structural integrity of Capillaries and have a definite role in wound healing.
- These tablets are very low cost and readily available.

9. No Antibiotics and Analgesics

The non-inclusions of these two key drugs is based on the evidences gathered over the time.

It has been observed and evidenced by serial pus culture that PRP induced healing have led to the control and cure of infections in the wounds.

The wounds positive for growth of Staphylococci, Pneumococci, Kliebsella etc have responded well to STARS therapy.

Significant observations regarding infections are:

- The MRSA positive wounds have responded very well, with no further need for any antibiotics. These wounds included postoperative burst abdomen wounds following Caesarean section too. (Figure 19 A, B)

- The wounds with pouring pus and discharge have healed without the need of any antibiotics. Rather their general well-being got built up as all antibiotics were stopped and STARS therapy started. (Figure 20 A, B)

- Wet gangrenous changes getting converted to dry within 2–3 sessions, including the Post-operative flap necrosis. (Figure 21 A, B). In such cases PRP is instilled under the flap.

  This action is also attributable to the antimicrobial properties of PRP and perhaps through inherent power of neo-angiogenesis to resist the infections, as is speculated in process of distraction osteogenesis, where the "infection is said to burn in the fire of regenerate".

How so ever as abundant precaution, weekly swab is taken from the wounds and send for culture and sensitivity till no growth is reported.

If at any point the infection seems to be worsening the appropriate drugs can be started.

Though till now we have very occasionally come across such scenario.

Most of these wounds have healed without further need of any antibiotics.

The only bacteria which have not responded so well is E.Coli.

The antibiotics for any other reasons/conditions/co-morbidities continues to be given.

Similarly, most of the patients did not required any analgesics on regular basis. This can only be speculated to be a added advantage of PRP therapy which promotes Proliferative inflammation rather than usual inflammatory cycle.

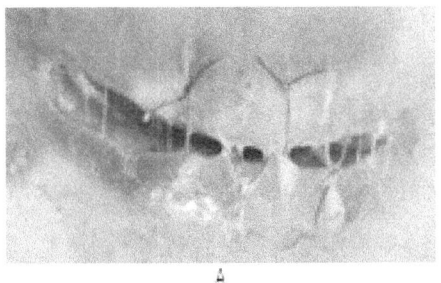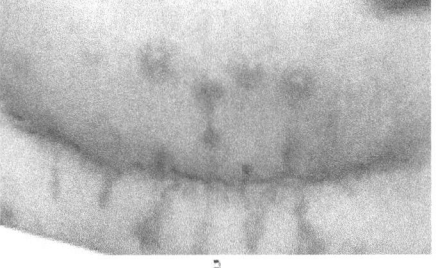

Figure 19: A: Showing pouring pus in compound fracture – MRSA positive
B. After 4 sessions: Complete infection Control.
C. After 8 sessions: Complete healing

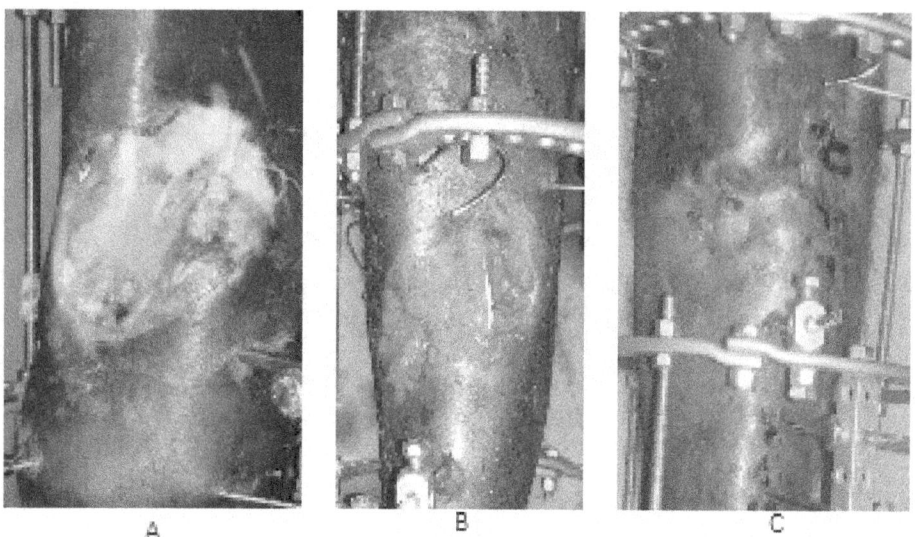

Figure 20: A: Showing a progressive postoperative flap necrosis with infection

B: After 2 sessions: Showing the damage restriction & limited to dry small superficial necrotic patch

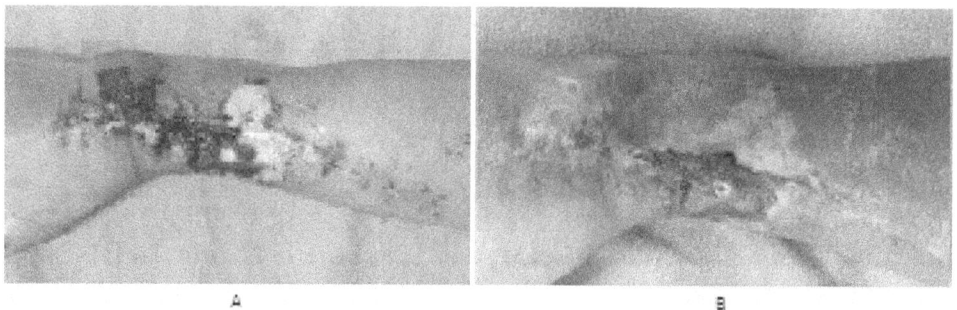

Figure 21: A: Showing a progressive postoperative flap necrosis with infection

B: After 2 sessions: Showing the damage restriction & limited to dry small superficial necrotic patch

10. No/Minimum Surgical Interventions

The STARS therapy obviates the need for surgical removal of damaged tissues for following Observations:

- The phagocytic activity is high after STARS therapy in the local tissue, particularly in very early phase. This leads to auto debridement's of the damaged, dead and necrotized tissue by the macrophages and there is no need for any mechanical removals of such tissue. As the infection is also well controlled simultaneously, hence such wounds with dead tissue do not pose for any further threat for septicemia or increase in infection.

- The tissue including skin flap, muscles, tendons and bone which seemed to be dead and necrotic, by naked eyes; are not totally devoid of vascularity and after few sessions of STARS they started showing red/pink spots/speckles of vascularity, and then healthy granulation covered them and eventually they survived. Only very minimal portion got necrotized to get separated as dry gangrene. (Figure 22 A, B,C)

- Large wounds healed completely with good skin coverage. almost scar less, not requiring surgery.

- The wounds with exposed underlying Orthopaedic implants such as plates, eventually got covered and healed, not requiring any removals.

- In wounds of foot with partial losses, the healing was obtained with Sole regeneration on plantar aspects and normal skin on dorsal aspect. This is a big leap in wound management as surgical sole transplantation/grafting is not possible due to morbidity of opposite side.

At the same time, it is observed that wounds which underwent debridement and later referred for STARS therapy, showed a remarkably fast recovery, with the whole wounds getting covered with healthy granulation tissue within 2 sessions as against usual 4-6 sessions. Perhaps this is due to bypassing the phase of "Suppression of unhealthy tissue", but comes with an irreversible loss of tissues which were surgically removed.

At this stage, its recommended that though no surgery is required effective treatment with STARS, but if need be;

- A debridement can be undertaken, avoiding the overzealous removal of any tissue or vital damaged tissues such tendons, as there is a fair chance that they would survive after treatment with STARS therapy.

- Similarly, for patient willing to undergo surgical skin grafting's etc, PRP infiltration in bed improves the outcomes.

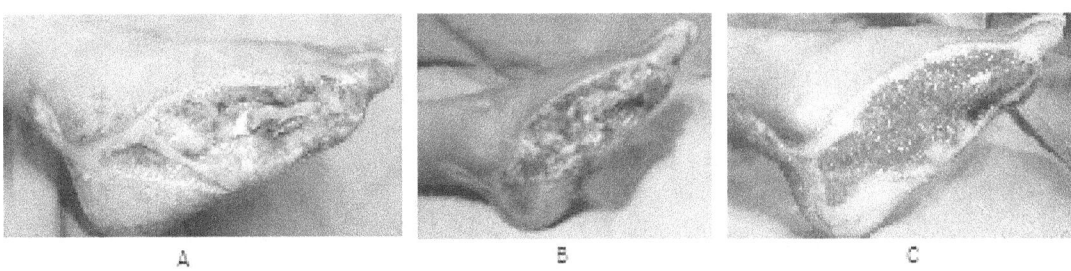

Figure: 22

The major advantage of this clinical protocol of STARS therapy are

- Wound management of the co-morbid/high risk patients suffering from diseases where drugs cannot be given like with renal failures, liver failures or heart failures.

- In the prevention of antimicrobial resistance. The successful development of wound management without the use of such antibiotics is a major step towards curtailment of antimicrobial resistance.

- Prevention of various risks due to antibiotics, which renders patient vulnerable to side effects/adverse events and their complications.

- Similarly, prevention of various risks of the analgesics particularly the renal failures etc.

- Adding to cost effectiveness, as both of these drugs are costly and are otherwise given for long durations. Hence a huge resource expenditure is saved by STARS therapy protocol.

- Negating the Surgical and Anesthesia risks in Patients, by obviating the need for surgery in wound management.

- Taking wound care to next level particularly by Sole regenerations and gangrene preventions, reversal and limitation.

The exclusion of need for drugs & intense surgery by STARS therapy, and reversal of gangrenous changes; are giant leap and paradigm shift from science of reconstruction to science of regeneration.

5

Problems/Difficulties and Complications

Following problems/difficulties/complications were observed with the STARS therapy:

- Pain during infiltration.

- Leakage and bursting of neo epithelized tissue

- Reluctance in blood withdrawals – too frequent due to 4th day protocol.

- New wounds & abscesses in near vicinity: Particularly in diabetic patients, though the primary wounds responded very well, were seen in some Patients, which needed I&D and further STARS therapy.

- Recurrence of wounds particularly in tropical foot ulcers,

  The partial regain of sensation were not enough for doing away with protective foot wears. (Figure 23 A, B, C)

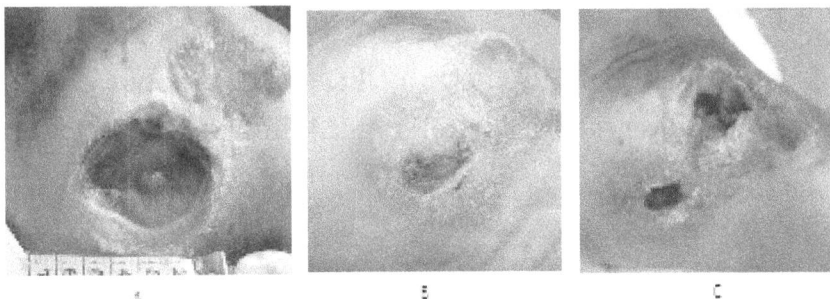

Figure 23: A: Showing Trophical Ulcer over foot.

B: Complete healing.

C: Recurrence after 4 months and a new ulcer after faulty Foot wear usage.

6

Pathology of Wound Healing
by STARS Therapy

A. Gross Pathology & Stages of wound healing

The wound grossly shows typical pattern of healing. This pattern can be staged into four stages/

    I. **Stage of Suppression of Unhealthy tissue**

   II. **Stage of Heathy Granulation**

 III. **Stage of Defect leveling and progression of epithelization**

 IV. **Stage of maturation of Epithelization**

I. **The stage of suppression of unhealthy tissue** is basically initial process led by Phagocytes where in auto debridement and infection control is triggered after PRP infiltrations.

This is stage where in the body starts limiting the damages.

The two key changes are:

- The damaged tissues start showing a sign of life including appearance of speckles of neo angiogenesis inside and over them. (Figure 24 A, B.) This is seen particularly in acute wounds.

- The floor of wound becomes pink and margins also starts showing regeneration and become pinkish. (Figure 25 A, B)

- The infection starts regressing. In cases of Gangrenes this is seen as wet gangrene getting converted into dry gangrene.

- Mostly in this stage the patient pains also start lowering down to minimal levels.

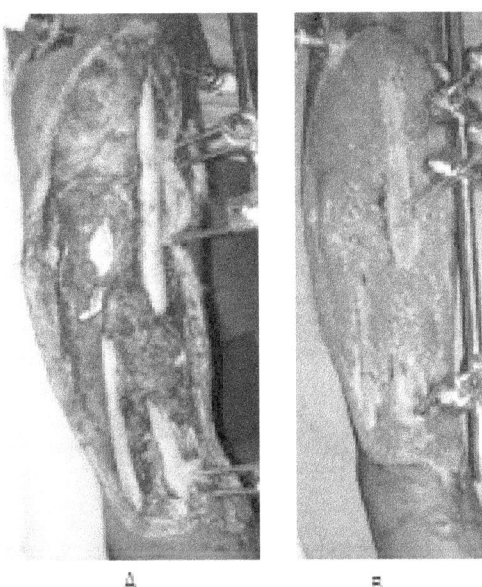

Figure 24: A: Showing exposed Muscles of Leg & Tibia bone: Developing necrosis
B: The Stage of Suppression of Unhealthy tissue: Showing the appearance of
speckles of angiogenesis in muscles and bone.

II.   **Stage of Healthy granulation:** In this stage, neo-angiogenesis takes place and covers the whole wound. This is the beginning of Proliferative inflammation/healing.

The key changes are: (Figure 25 C)

- Appearance of health bright red granulation in the wound.
- The whole floor is covered by the same
- The exposed tissues such as tendons, bones are also covered by the granulation.
- Mostly as this stage is reached the infections are well controlled
- The margins start showing a bit of progression from periphery of wound towards center.

III.   **Stage of Defect – Filling:** In this stage, the granulation tissue levels up and fills the depth of the wound.

The key changes are: (Figure 25 D)

- Appearance of uniform red healthy granulation tissue
- Levelling up of the granulation to the neo-epithelizing wound margins
- Shrinking of wound.
- The skin starts regenerating from the periphery.
- Eventually by the end of this stage the skin will regenerate and cover the whole wound.

IV. **Stage of Maturation of Epithelization:** This is final stage for wound healing. The regenerated skin will cover the whole wound and mature to near normal texture and elasticity. An almost scar less healing wound be witnessed at the end.

The key changes are: (Figure 25E)

- The pinkish fragile neo-epithelize skin will mature gradually.
- This skin is mostly of near normal character matching to the adjoining one.
- The sole will regenerate with sole-characteristic.
- This stage is overlapping with previous ones, so as the neo-epithelization forms,
- the older one starts maturating.
- The matured skin is rich in fibro-collagen tissue.
- This is usually the longest stage of healing.

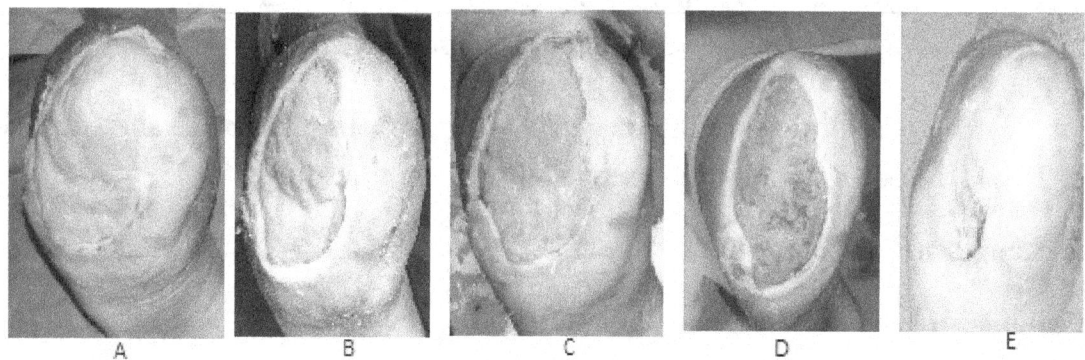

Figure 25: A: Showing infected chronic non-healing diabetic ulcer of foot

B. Showing Stage I – Suppression of Unhealthy tissue with pink floor and margins.

C. Showing Stage II – Healthy Granulation: Appearance and covering of floor by healthy granulation tissue.

D. Showing Stage III – Defect-Filling: The healthy granulation tissue levels with progressing neo-epithelizing regenerating skin and wound have started shrinking.

E. Showing Stage IV – Maturation of Epithelization: In this case the regenerated epithelization matured to Sole-Skin.

B. Histological Features

The histological features as seen through the progression of wound healing by STARS therapy are as following: (Figure 26 A, B, C, D)

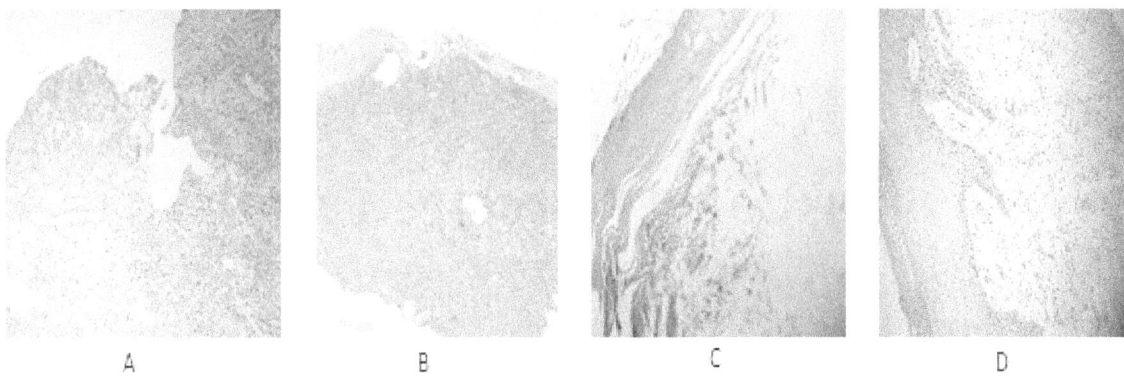

Figure 26: A: After 48 hours: Showing the wound defect with Phagocytic concentration along the margin.

B: After 10 days: Defect filling with Angiotic tissue.

C: After 21 days: Showing Complete filling up of defect with Collagen tissue.

D: After 6 weeks: Showing full thickness matured collagen led complete healing.

To Summarize, the pathology of healing process by PRP led STRAS therapy is typically Proliferative healing.

It assists the regeneration skin led by fibro-collagen tissue towards complete wound healing.

7

Illustrated Prototype Cases

A. Acute Injury Leading to Complex Wounds

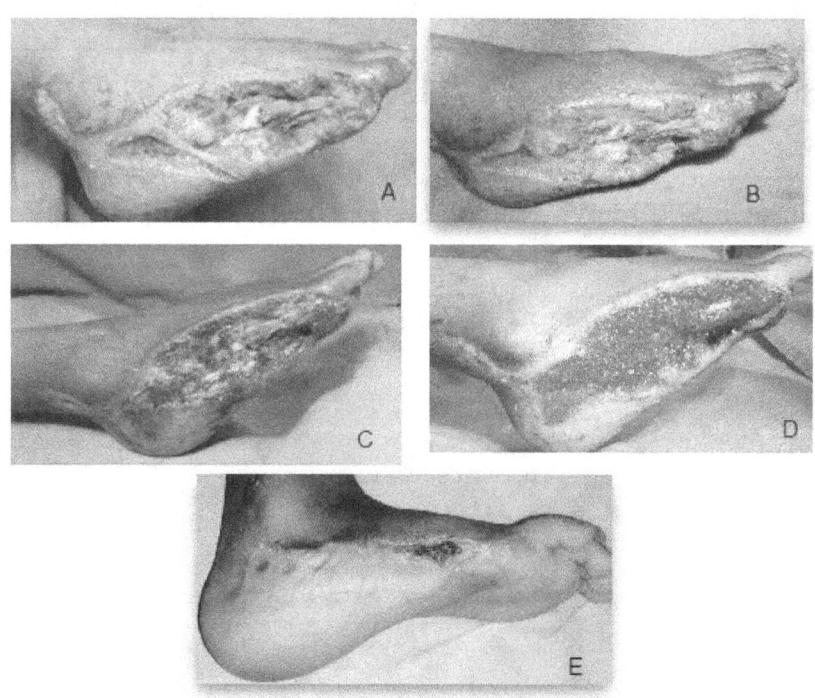

Figure:27: A. After Injury: exposed bones and tendon with necrosis.

B. After 2 sessions.

C. After 4 sessions.

D. After 6 sessions.

E: Full healing after 10 sessions.

1. 4 years old child, run over injury leading to partial loss of lateral aspect of foot

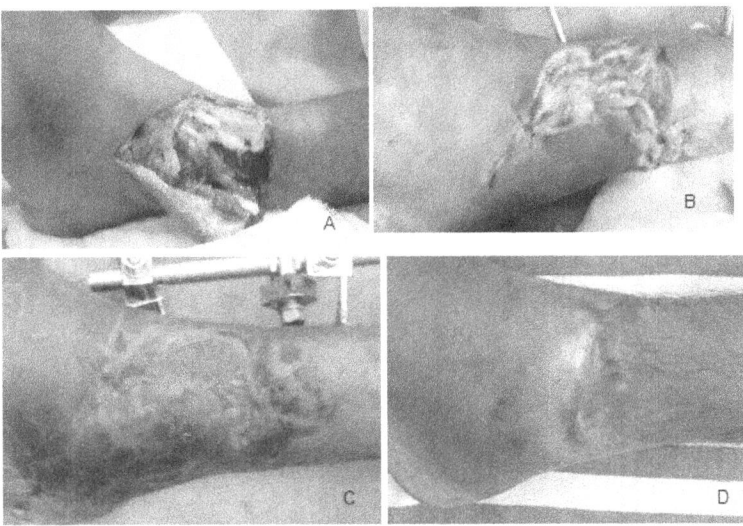

Figure 28: A. 5 days old injury – tendons showing necrosis.

B. After repair of tendons & stabilization.

C. After 4 sessions.

D. Complete healing after 6 sessions.

2. 33 years old Man sustained wound in road traffic accident – Compound fracture with exposed cut tendons with loss of skin.

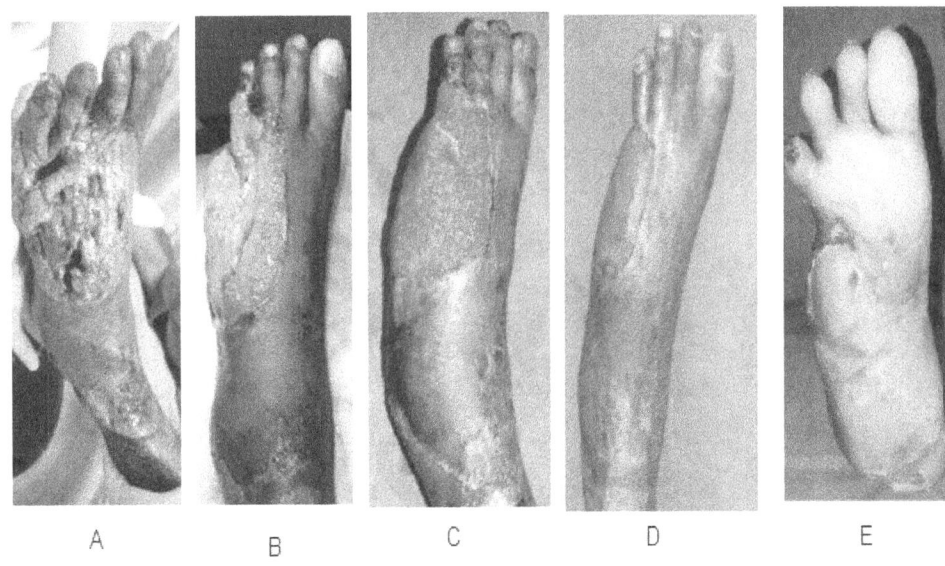

Figure 29: A. After injury.

B. After 3 sessions.

C, D: Granulation tissue filling up the defects along with shaping of foot.

E: Near complete recovery with regeneration of Sole & dorsal skins: after 12 sessions

3. Foot Reconstruction: 28 year old man sustained injury after road traffic accident, leading to Mangled extremity with loss of 4 metatarsal and 5 phalanges

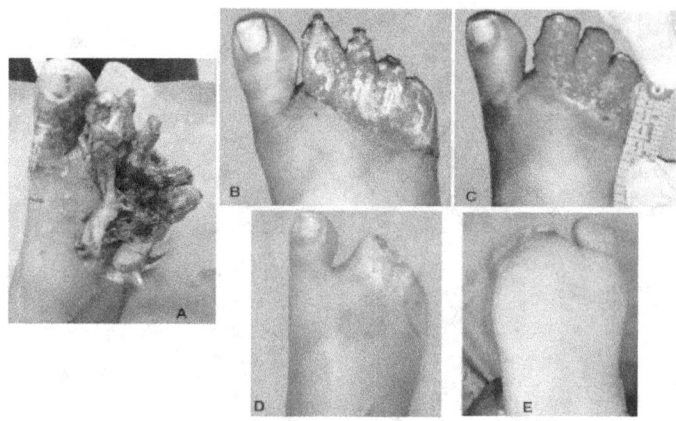

Figure 30: A. After Injury.

B. After 3 sessions – PRP is given at the base of wound on both side

C. Healthy Granulation tissue covering the bones

D & E: Skin regenerated over exposed toe covering all of them together.

4. A Mangled distal foot with all bones exposed and severe tissue loss

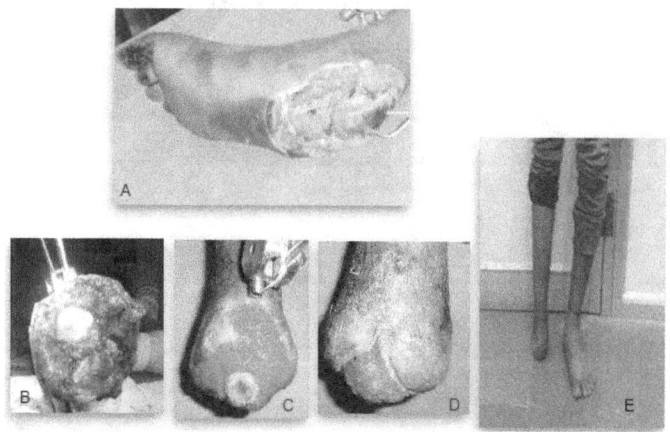

Figure 31: A. 10 days After injury: Exposed necrotizing Calcaeneum.
Developed Gas Gangrene of forefoot

B. After forefoot amputation

C. After 2 sessions

D. After 4 sessions

E. Complete wound healing and full weight bearing on regenerated stump
after 8 sessions

5. 22 years Male: Developed gas gangrene after injury of leg and foot

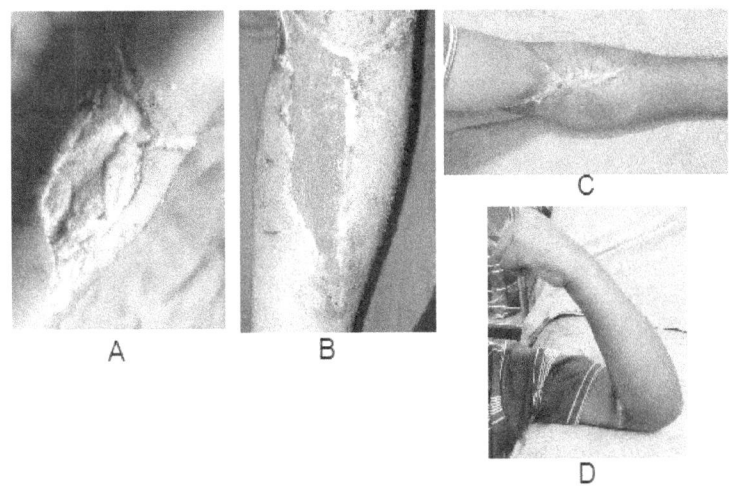

Figure 32: A: Infected wound over the elbow and forearm (Prone for difficult healing as wound crosses the joint)

B. After 4 sessions -Good health granulation with regeneration of skin and shrinking of wound C& D: Complete healing with full movements at elbow.

6. **38 years male: upper limb injury, a deep wound with infection extending across the elbow.**

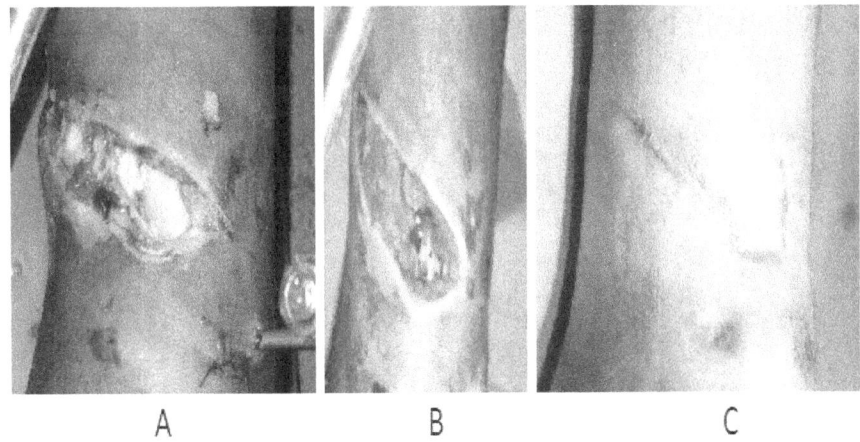

Figure 33: A. After stabilization – Exposed tibia and tendons with mild infection.

B. After 3 sessions- showing healthy granulation with control of Infection.

C. Complete healing after 7 sessions.

7. **28 years old male: compound fracture of tibia with exposed bone and tendon.**

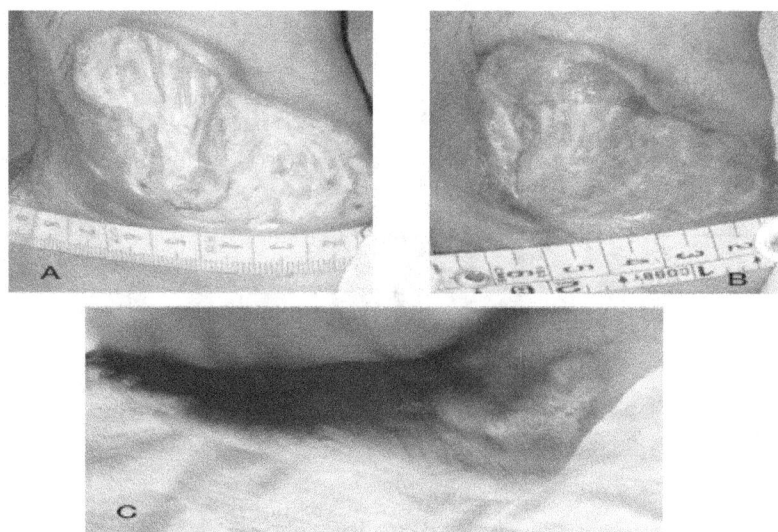

Figure 34: A. Venous ulcer over lateral malleolus, with exposed and sloughing tendon.

B. After 3 sessions -Tendon showing signs of Regeneration and Angiogenesis

C. Complete Recover after 8 sessions.

8. 55 years old Female:7 years old Venous ulcer over lateral aspect of lower leg and ankle.

B. Chronic Non-Healing Wounds

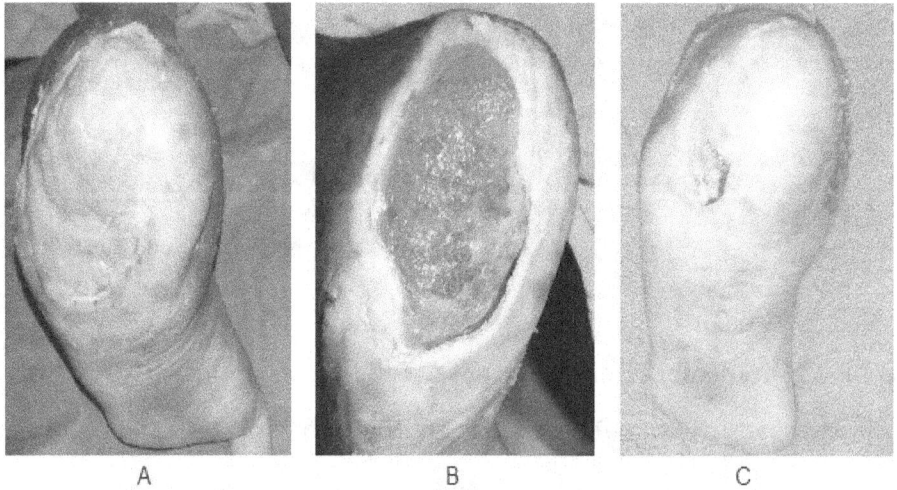

Figure 35: A. Long standing ulcer over heel with severe infection

**B. After 6 sessions of STAR Therapy filled up with healthy
granulation & regenerating skin margins.**

C. Complete healing after 10 sessions with Sole regeneration.

9. 22 years female – 5 years old Non-healing ulcer with juvenile diabetes & uncontrolled
    Sugar level.

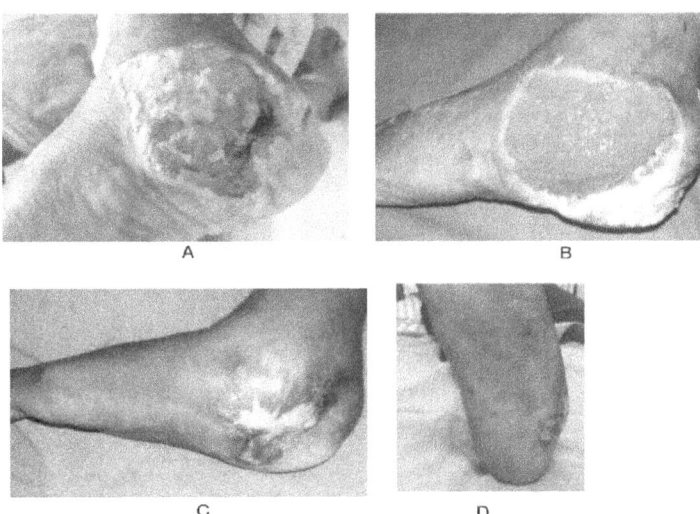

Figure 36: A. Severely infected wound with partial loss of heel.

B. After 6 sessions complete control of infection & healthy granulation.

C & D. Completely healed wound after 11 sessions.

10. 72 years Male: Non- healing with Chronic osteomyelitis of Calcaeneum with diabetes

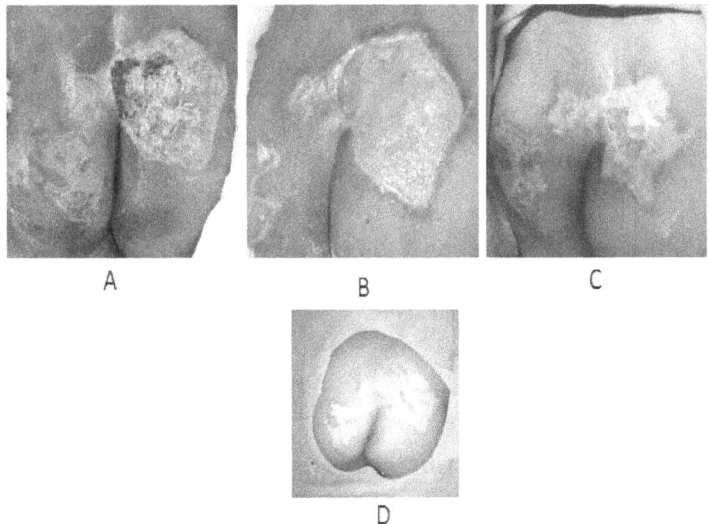

Figure 37: A. A progressive Grade IV bed sore – with exposed sacrum bone and infection.

B. After 4 sessions healthy granulation with regeneration of skin, control of infection

C. Nearly complete healing at the end if treatment after 7 sessions.

D. Completely healed after 11 sessions.

11. 65 years female: Bed sore, following prolonged immobilization due to Polytrauma, with diabetes.

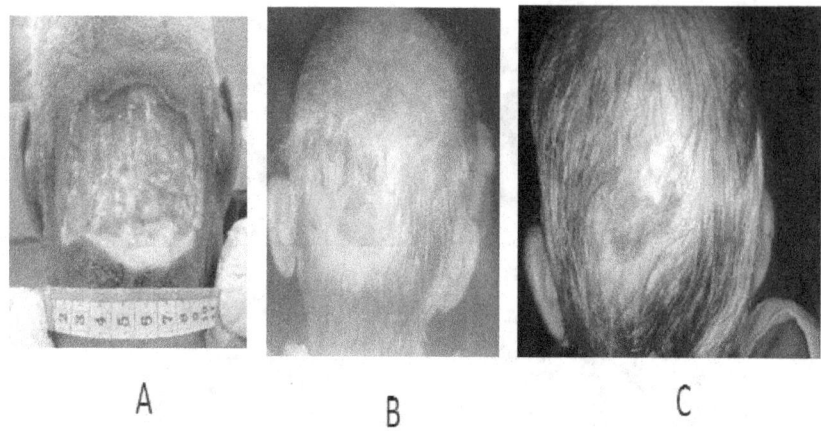

Figure 38: A. A Large Pressure ulcer over occiput exposing the skull.

B. After 4 session – healthy granulation, control of infection & good regeneration of skin.

C. At the end of treatment with complete healing after 6 sessions.

12. 45 years male: Infected Pressure sore over skull after prolong Coma.

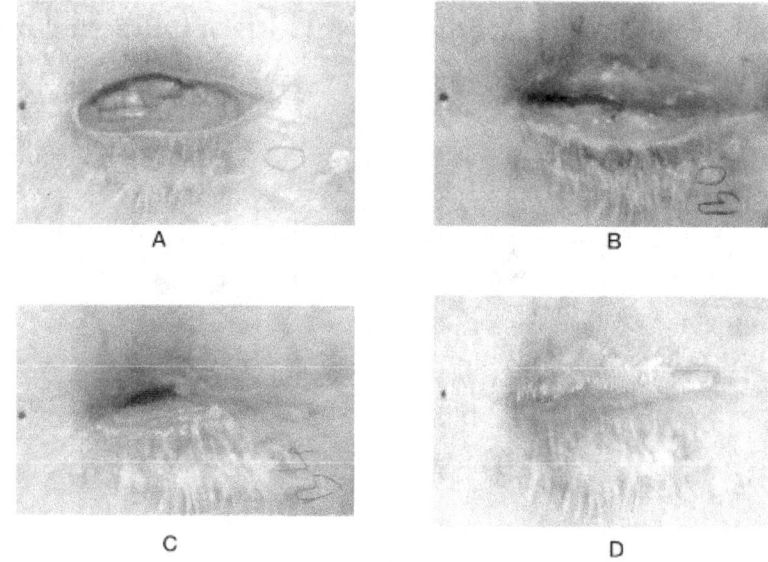

Figure 39: A. Deep wound with exposed spinal compression.

B. After 2 sessions: Infection control and health granulation

C. Good healing after 4 sessions

D. Complete healing after 6 sessions.

13. 65 years old female with diabetes – Non-healing Wound after spinal decompression.

C. Postoperative Wounds

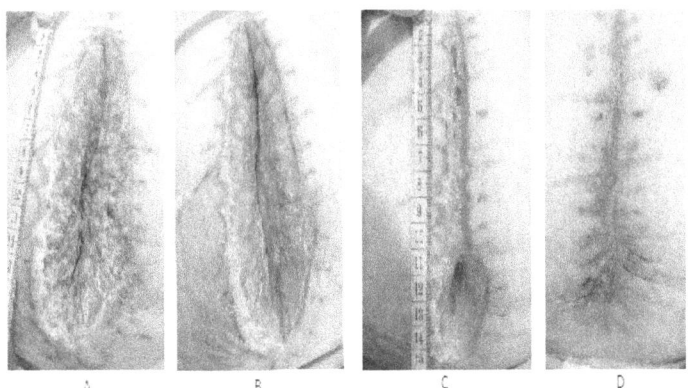

Figure 40: A. Infected abdominal – wound Dehiscence – 21 days after Surgery.

B. After 3 sessions – Control of infection and healthy granulation.

C. After 6 sessions.

D. Near complete healing after 8 sessions.

14. 42 years old female – Wound dehiscence after Hysterectomy

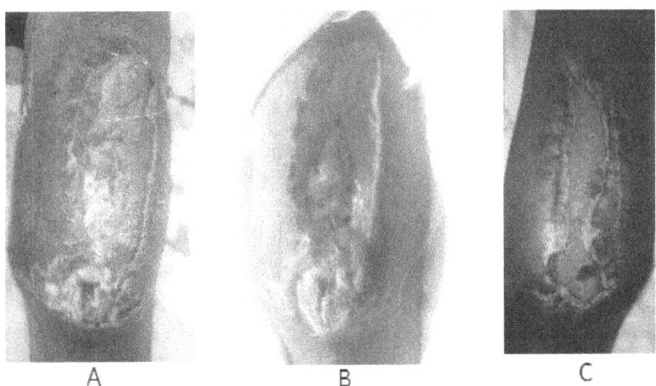

Figure 41: A. Wound with Exposed Patella, Wires over Patella and Patellar tendon.

B. After 4 sessions: Control of infection, healthy granulation tissue

C. Near complete healing with coverage of Bone, Implants and Tendon.

15. 27 years old male - Postoperative following skin flap necrosis exposing the underneath implants.

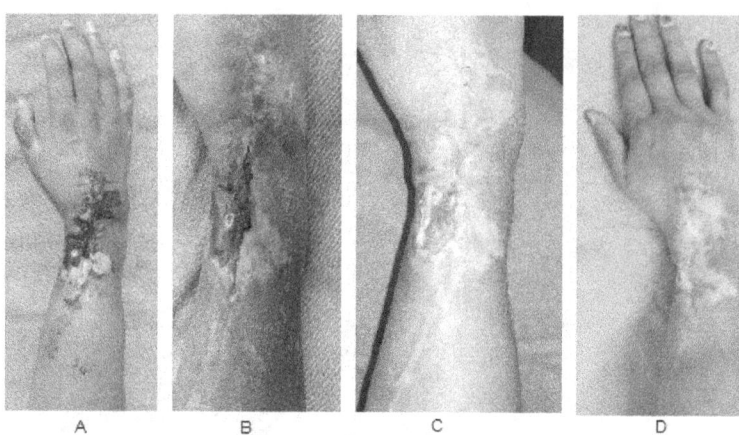

Figure 42: A. Necrosis of Major part of Flap with Infection.

B. After 2 sessions: The Infection is controlled and flap necrosis is limited, with regeneration of remaining part

C. Spontaneous removal of superficial necrosed flap. Complete Healing: After 6 sessions.

16. 29 years female: After Giant Cell Tumor removal of distal radius - Flap necrosis

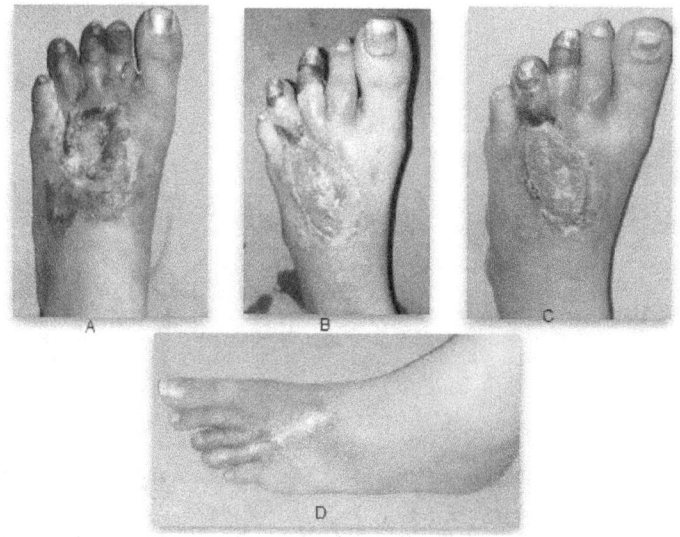

Figure 43: A. Injury leading to necrosis of skin flap and gangrenous changes in III & IV Toe

B, C: During treatment: The gangrenous changes limited to distal most part and wound showing healthy granulation

D. Complete healing with salvage of both the Toes, after 8 sessions.

17. 18 years old girl: Developing gangrene of toes and flap necrosis, after sustaining injury in road traffic accident.

D. Damage Control in Gangrene

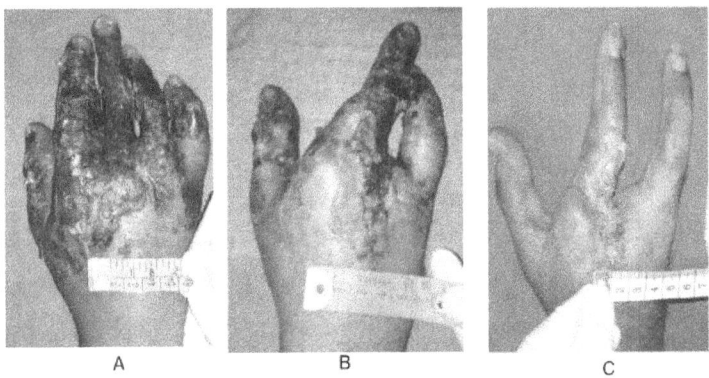

Figure 44: A. Hand showing gangrenous changes in all fingers.

B. The middle and ring fingers could not be saved but rest are showing improvements

C. All the other fingers are salvaged and functional, after 7 sessions.

18. 62 years Male: Severe infection of hand with gangrenous changes in all fingers, with Uncontrolled Diabetes.

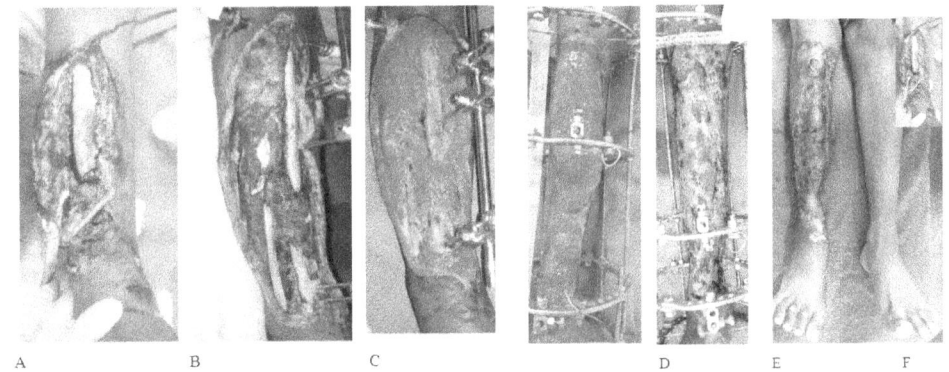

Figure 45: A. After injury with bone loss and necrosis particularly of distal tibia.

B. After debridement and stabilization.

C. After 4 sessions: Showing regeneration in bone and wound.

D. After 10 sessions: Showing complete coverage with Granulation and Skin regeneration.

E. Healing of wound (Distraction- Osteogenesis was done for bone loss).

F. Complete Healing after 29 sessions.

19. 15 years boy – Compound type III C (Gustilo & Anderson) fracture with bone loss of tibia

E. Limb Salvage

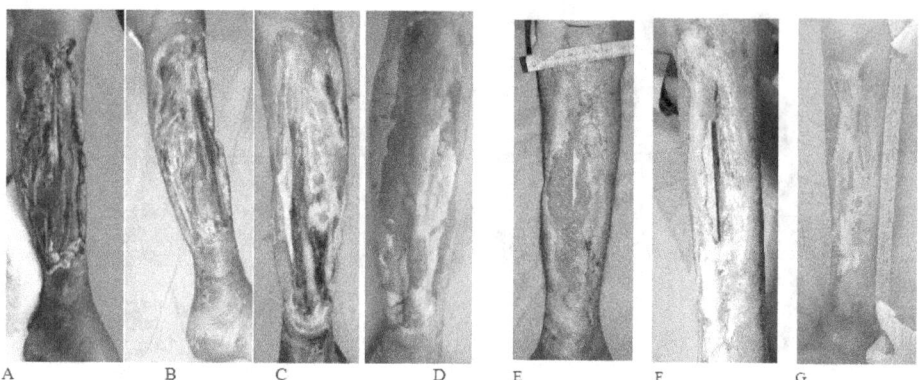

Figure 46: A: Showing complete necrosis of muscles and bone, after fasciotomy.

B. C, D: During Treatment: Showing regeneration through angiogenesis in all tissue.

E: After 14 sessions: Showing health granulation in the wound & skin regeneration.

F. After 18 sessions the treatment was discontinued with exposed Fibula, which got Sequestrated.

G. Complete Healing: He resumed the treatment and Sequestrated fibular was removed & wound healed Spontaneously.

20. 52 years Male: Gangrene of leg following compartment syndrome.

F. Reversal of Near Gangrene

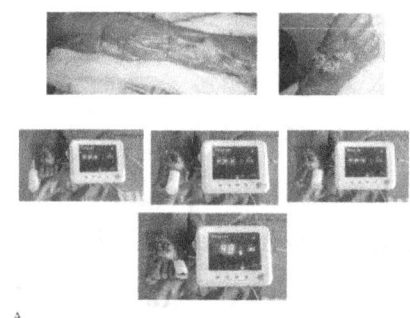

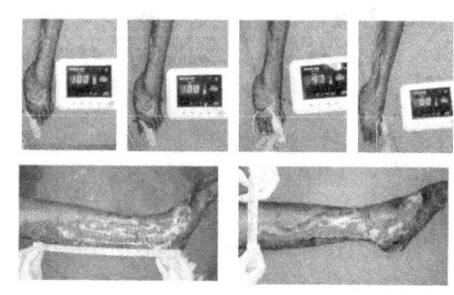

Figure 47: A. After injury: No capillary circulation, Dorsalis Paedis and SpO2 in toes, except little toes

Figure 47: B. After 4 sessions: Regeneration led to improvement in capillary and collateral circulations, leading to return of SpO2 in most of toes, and healing of wound.

21. 57 years Female: 2 days old road traffic injury with loss of skin and soft tissues with vascular deficit.

Chapter IV

PRP for Tendinopathies

1

Introduction

PRP therpy focuses upon Implantation **into a site of damage/healing. Role in regenerating tissue and producing growth factors** is important in the healing process. Cells maintain their pluripotency following transplantation and undergo site-specific differentiation. Differentiate into Endothelial cells, Osteoblasts, and Fibroblasts Act as a "Biologic Patch" and this augment the healing process through the increased production of collagen and proteoglycan, particularly in case of tendons.

Structure of Tendon and Changes in Tendinopathy

They consist of primarily of WATER & TYPE I COLLAGEN and Cells- fibroblasts. Extracellular matrix (ECM):

a. Tenoblasts and Tenocytes.

- o 90–95% of the cellular elements of tendons.
- o 5–10% – chondrocytes, synovial cells of the tendon sheath
- o and vascular cells including capillary endothelial cells & smooth muscle cells of arteriole.

b. Glycosaminoglycans (GAG), glycoproteins and several other small molecules.

Adhesive Proteoglycanslycoproteins such as fibronectin and thrombospondin, participate in repair and regenerative processes in tendon.

Tenascin-C, another important component of the tendon ECM, is abundant in the tendon body, osteotendinous (OTJ) and myotendinous (MTJ) junctions.

c. Collagen is arranged in hierarchical levels of increasing complexity, beginning with tropocollagen which is triple-helix polypeptide chain.

It unites into fibrils; fibers (primary bundles); fascicles (secondary bundles); tertiary bundles and the tendon itself.

The structure changes are classically described by following two classifications:

Clancy's Classification for Tendinopathy

Minor repeated trauma leads to degeneration.

There are 3 stages, which a tendinopathy undergoes (Figure):

a. Tenosynovitis

b. Tendonitis

c. Tendinosis

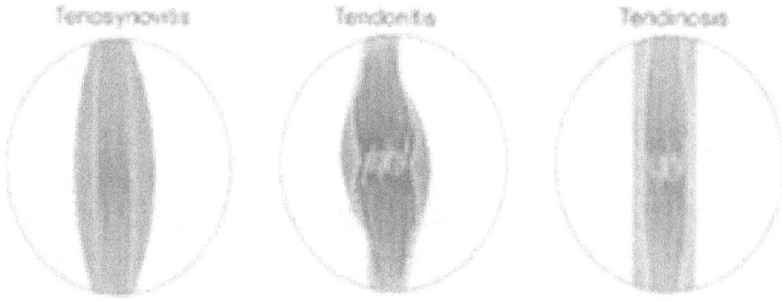

Figure 48: Showing Clnacy's Classification for Tendinopathy
(Courtesy reference)

Bonar's Modification of Clancy's Classification

a. Tendinosis:

- Intratendinous degeneration (commonly due to ageing, micro-trauma).
- Collagen disorientation, disorganisation and fibre separation by an increase in mucoid ground substance,
- Increased prominence of cells and vascular spaces with or without neovascularization and focal necrosis or calcification

b. Tendinitis/Partial rupture:

- Symptomatic degeneration of the tendon with vascular disruption and inflammatory repair response

- Degenerative changes as noted above with superimposed evidence of tear, including fibroblastic and myofibroblastic proliferation, haemorrhage and organizing granulation tissue.

c. Paratenonitis:

'Inflammation' of the outer layer of the tendon (paratenon) alone, whether or not the paratenon is lined by synovium

d. Paratenonitis with tendinosis:

- Paratenonitis associated with intratendinous degeneration

- Degenerative changes as noted in tendinosis with mucoid degeneration with or without fibrosis and scattered inflammatory cells in the paratenon alveolar tissue.

2

Rationale

The cellular phase of tendon healing is depicted in the Figure 8.

The 3 phases of inflammation, proliferation and Remodelling.

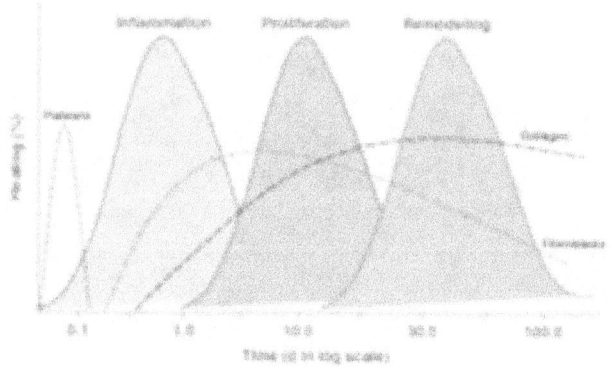

Figure 49: Showing the Cellular phase of Tendon healing

The following table 4 describes the day wise changes in the tendon after injury

0	Immediately post injury	Clot formation around the wound
0-1	Inflammatory	First battery of growth factors and inflammatory molecules produced by cells within the blood clot
1-2	Inflammatory	Invasion by extrinsic cells, phagocytosis
2-4	Proliferative	Further invasion by extrinsic cells followed by second battery of growth factors that stimulate fibroblast proliferation
4-7	Reparative	Collagen deposition, granulation tissue formation, revascularization
7-14	Reparative	Injury site becomes more organized, extracellular matrix is produced in large amounts

| 14-21 | Remodelling | Decreases in cellular and vascular content, increases in collagen type I |
| 21+ | Remodelling | Collagen continues to become more organized and cross-linked with healthy matrix outside the injury area. Collagen ratios, water content and cellularity begin to approach normal levels |

Table 4: Showing day-wise changes during tendon repair.

a. **Inflammatory phase (one week after injury):**

- Fibroblasts and macrophages from extrinsic and intrinsic sources migrate to the site of injury.

- The primary events include phagocytosis of clot and necrotic tissue and deposition of extracellular matrix.

b. **Fibroblastic phase (three weeks after injury):**

- There is proliferation of fibroblasts at the injury site.

- The primary events of this phase are deposition of collagen at the site of injury and revascularization.

c. **Remodelling phase (eight weeks after injury):**

- Newly produced collagen fibre becomes organised linearly along the axis of the tendon.

- Adhesions between the tendon and the sheath become more pronounced

Changes at Molecular Levels

The inflammatory pathway is through secretion of growth factors, including

- Platelet-derived growth factor (PDGF),

- Transforming growth factor-Î± and -Î2 (TGF-Î±, TGF-Î2),

- Fibroblast growth factor (bFGF), and Epidermal growth factor (EGF).

These growth factors lead to

- direct the attraction and proliferation of fibroblasts and

- stimulate collagen and protein synthesis.

The Fibroblasts play the central role in healing and remodelling tendon at the site of injury.

This process takes considerable time, and even at maturation, the biomechanical properties of healed tissue are inferior to those of uninjured tendon due to a complicated system including a proportional decrease in the amount of collagen I and an increase in the amount of collagen III

The Cytokines present in the PRP can be targets for tissue engineering. Engineered tissue can be created by:

- Altering the responding cells,

- Augmenting the healing signals,

- Blocking the inhibitor pathways, or creating de novo tissue in a bioreactor,

- Manipulating with signalling molecules in the correct biomechanical environment to form a tendon.

3

Key Evidence in Literature

- 2006: G Banfi et al: PRP in tendinopathies of professional athletes.

  - Statistically significant change in EGF and CCL_2. VEGF concentrations were high.

- 2007: Mikel Sanchez et al: The effect of autologous platelet-rich matrices during Achilles tendon surgery for promoting healing and functional recovery. "Recovered their range of motion earlier, showed no wound complication and took less time to take up gentle running and to resume training activities.

- 2008: Marieke de Moset et al: Performed a cell culture study to prove that platelet-rich plasma has a positive effect on cell proliferation and collagen production. PRCR, but also PPCR, stimulates cell proliferation and total collagen production.

- 2008: Yoshiteru Kajikawa et al: Locally injected PRP is useful as an activator of circulation-derived cells for enhancement of initial tendon healing process.

- 2008: Steven Sampson et al reviewed literature on PRP therapy and summarised that PRP provides a promising alternative to surgery by promoting safe and natural healing. However, there are only few controlled trials and he concluded that as clinical use increases.

- 2009: Allan Mishra emphasised that not only acute tendon injuries, chronic tendinitis may also benefit with PRP injections. Specifically, it could be possible to treat an acute Achilles tendon tear non-operatively using a PRP injection

- 2010: Jianying Zhang et al results indicated that PRCR treatment induced differentiation of TSCs into activated tenocytes. Enhances tendon healing, as tenocytes induced to differentiate, Proliferate quickly and produce abundant collagen to repair injured tendons.

- 2010: Giuseppe Longo et al did a systemic review on tissue engineered biological augmentation for tendon healing by performing a comprehensive search of PubMed, Medline, Cochrane, CINAHL and Embase databases:"several new techniques are available but there was a lack of definite conclusion and emphasized on the need for detailed study"

- 2011: Roslyn T Nguyen et al: application of platelet rich plasma in Musculoskeletal and Sports medicine and concluded Platelet rich plasma have a positive augmentative effect on tendon healing.

- 2011 Paolin: There is a lack of high-level evidence regarding randomized clinical trials assessing the efficacy of PRP treating ligament and tendon injuries. "The potential risks involved with PRP are fortunately very low. However, benefits remain unproven to date

- 2013 Nikolas Baksh: performed a systematic review of the basic science literature on the use of platelet-rich plasma (PRP) in tendon models. 8 in vivo studies found decreased tendon repair time, increased fibre organization or both.8 in vitro studies reported that PRP treatment increased cell proliferation; 7 reported an increase in growth factor expression. 3 in vivo studies found increased vascularity and 4 found increased tensile strength.

  However, he concluded that literature was inconsistent with regard to reporting the methods of preparation of PRP and in reporting platelet concentrations and cytology.

- Currently PRP is administered to almost 86,000 athletes in the United States and Europe to treat acute and chronic tendon, ligament, and muscle injuries. Because of its wide spread use, it is estimated that the market value of PRP will reach $126 million

4

Our Experience

We have conducted many studies regarding effect of PRP in tendon healing. The key ones are - in acute injuries, in Rabbit Model and for supraspinatus tendonitis. Also for clinical benefits in tennis elbow. A summary of the findings is as following:

A. Preclinical Evidence of PRP Usage in Tendon Healing

Acute Injuries – Rabbit Model.

We conducted animal model study for building evidence on tendon healing with PRP usage, in 2009-11.

The experiment included study of natural tendon healing Vs PRP induced healing in TA.

The left forefoot and hind foot were in control Group and Right Fore foot and Hind foot were PRP induced healing.

The forefoot tendons were acutely repaired, whereas in hind foot a gap of 10mm was created, the defect was left alone in Control group whereas in PRP group it was bridged with PRP soaked Bio-absorbable gel and tendon sheath was repaired over it.

The Table 5 Summarizes the key findings.

The Figure 50 A, B, C, D shows the sequential histological changes in control group and Figure 51A, B, C, D shows in PRP groups. The healing was predominantly fibro-collagenous led in case of PRP group, including in bridging the tendon defect. These Key findings are summarized in graphic manner in Figure 52A, B, C, D.

The PRP have led to filling up of defects in near normal manner as was seen in primary repair, including bridging the defect of about 10mm, when used along a biological scaffold.

This gives us insight and evidence that in rupture intra-lesional PRP should lead to good healing.

S N	Name	Weeks after procedure	Left forefoot Control foot Percutaneous tenotomy without prp	Right forefoot Experimental foot Percutaneous tenotomy - with prp	Left hindfoot Control foot With 10mm gap - without prp	Right hindfoot Experimental foot With 10mm gap - with prp
1	Rabbit A	3 weeks	Myocytolysis with sparse chronic non-specific inflammatory infiltrate. Sparse granulation tissue formation	Tissue show evidence of myocytolysis with few regenerated myocytes and non specific chronic inflammatory infiltrate with granulation tissue formation	Tissue shows predominantly fibro-collagenous tissue with unremarkable myocytes and sparse inflammatory infiltrate	Tissue shows evidence of myocyte regeneration with fibrotic tissue elements. Chronic non specific infiltrate and granulation tissue formation
	Impression:		Minimal evidence of healing. Non specific inflammation	Early evidence of healing	Evidence of healing by secondary intention	Evidence of granulation tissue formation- early healing present
2	Rabbit B	6 weeks	Tissue shows evidence of myocytolysis with non-specific chronic inflammatory infiltrate (focal). Minimal granulation tissue formation	Evidence of extensive fibrotic tissue elements with foreign body giant cell reaction. Granulation tissue formation seen	Tissue shows evidence of extensive fibrotic tissue changes with foreign body giant cell reaction with myocyte degeneration	Tissue shows evidence of myocyte regeneration with fibrous tissue elements and granulation tissue formation
	Impression:		Early evidence of healing	Evidence of healing present	Evidence of healing by secondary intention	Evidence of healed fibrotic granulation tissue
3	Rabbit C	12 weeks	Predominantly fibro-collagenous tissue with non specific chronic inflammation with giant cell reaction. Myocytolysis with granulation tissue formation.	Tissue shows evidence of myocytolysis with regeneration of myocyte. There is evidence of granulation tissue formation	Tissue shows extensive fibro-collagenous tissue. Minimal evidence of granulation tissue formation	Tissue shows evidence of fibro-collagenous tissue with granulation tissue formation
	Impression:		Partial healing with granulation tissue	Evidence of healing present	Evidence of healing by secondary intention	Evidence of healing with granulation tissue
4	Rabbit D	16 weeks	Tissue shows evidence of myocytolysis with few fibres showing regenerative changes. Moderate amount of chronic inflammatory infiltrate seen with fibrous tissue formation	Tissue shows predominantly fibrocollagenous tissue with sparse amount of chronic inflammatory infiltrate. Presence of suture granuloma. Mild granulation tissue seen	Tissue shows predominantly extensive fibrocollagenous tissue with foreign body giant cell reaction (suture granuloma) with non specific chronic inflammatory infiltrate	Tissue shows fibrocollagenous tissue with evidence of granulation tissue formation with muscle fibre regeneration
	Impression:		Evidence of healing present	Evidence of healing with granulation tissue.	Evidence of healing with secondary intention	Evidence of healing with granulation tissue formation

Table 5: Showing the Evidence of Tendon healing by PRP in Rabbit.

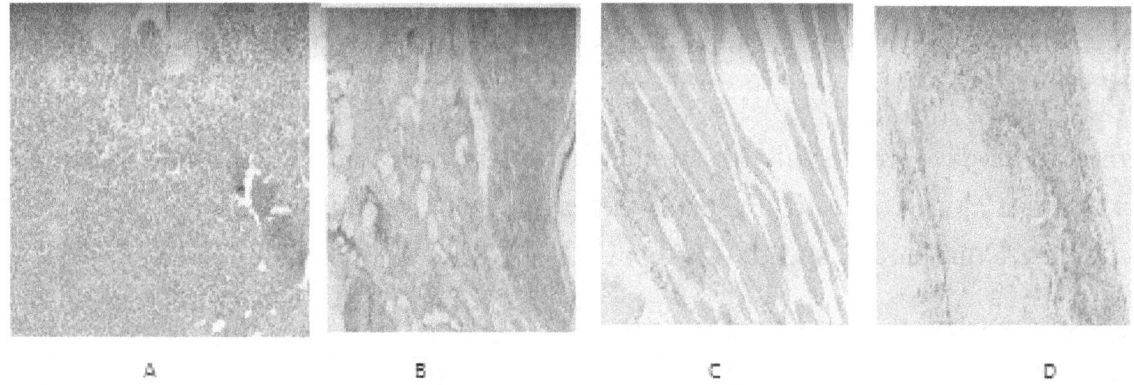

A   B   C   D

Figure 50: A: Left forefoot at 3 weeks – Inflammatory Response

B: Left forefoot at 12 weeks – Inflammatory Cells and Granulation tissue

C: Left hind foot at 3 Weeks: Sparse Inflammatory cells and Fibrous Tissue

D: left Hind foot at 12 weeks: Inflammatory infiltrate granulation tissue with Fibrous tissue

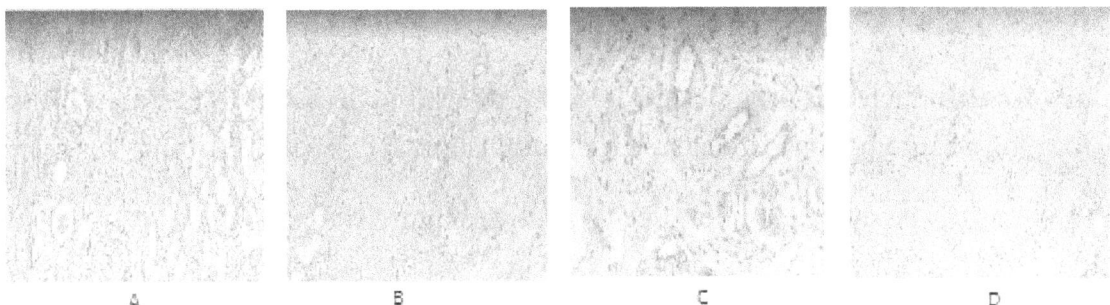

Figure 51: A: Right forefoot at 3 weeks: Inflammatory infiltrate and granulation tissue with Myocytes regeneration

B: Right forefoot at 12 weeks: Fibro-collagenase tissue.

C: Right Hind foot at 3 weeks: Fibro-collagenase tissue

D: Right Hind foot: Fibro –collagenase tissue.

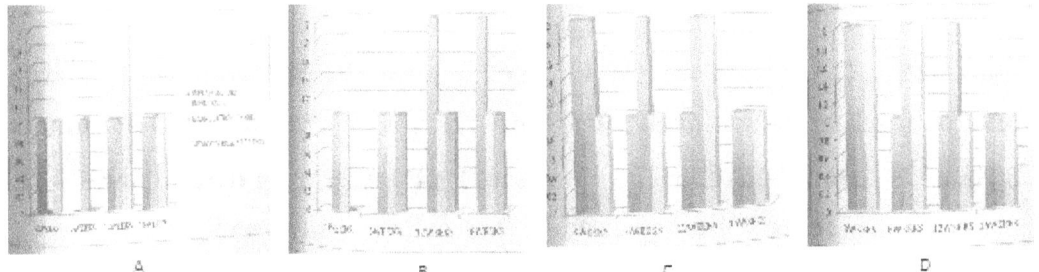

Figure 52: A. Left Fore foot – Primary repair.

B. Left Hind foot – Defect 10mm

C: PRP induced healings in primary repair.

D: PRP induced healing in Gap.

Many other in vivo animal studies conclude that:

- 2 weeks PRP treatment increased load at failure by 72.2%, stress by 39.1%, and stiffness by 53.1% compared to untreated controls

- PRP treatment also induced better cell orientation and tissue maturation

- PRP could accelerate the tendon wound healing process

- PRP was also found to increase the expression of growth factors (IGF-I) in healed tendons

- Confirming the safety of PRP use in vivo.

Clinical Evidence At Our Centre

Another study was conducted as part of Ph.D by Dr. Pradeep Singh in looking into the clinical effects of local infiltration of autologous Platelet supernatant in supraspinatus tendinopathy

The key findings are as per the figure number 12 A, B and figure number 13.

The PRP infiltration led to fibro-collagenous healing

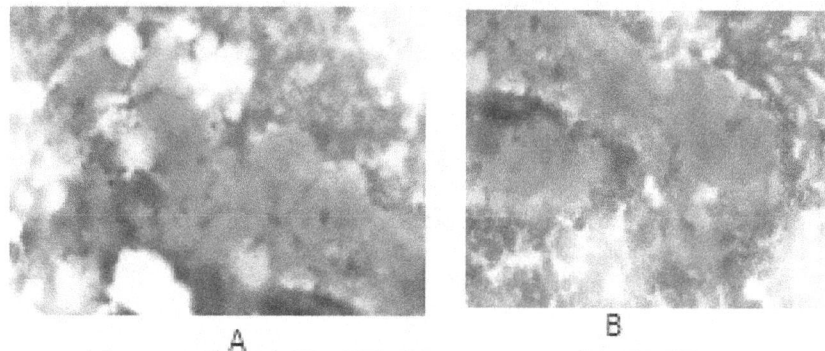

Figure 53*: A. Grade I lesion: FANC after 7 months of PRP infiltration: Tendon fibres with reacting tenosynovial cell activity along with fibro-collagenous material
B: Grade II lesion: FNAC after 8 months of PRP infiltration tendon fibres with reactive fibrocytes and Fibro-collagenous tissue
*courtesy Pradeep Singh

Practice at Our centre

Indications:

The PRP is being used for tendinopathies Rotator Cuff including supraspinatus tendonitis

- Tennis Elbow
- Plantar Fasciitis
- Tendo- Achilles tendonitis
- And other tendon and Ligament injuries such as Medical Collateral Ligament and Lateral collateral ligament f Knee.
- Augmentation of healing after reconstruction of Anterior cruciate ligaments

Eligible Patient's:

- Mostly with incomplete ruptures and intra-substance tear/lesion.
- No blood disorders/dyscarisis and with normal platelet counts.

Technique for Infiltration of PRP

It can be done under USG guidance or directly in the lesion through clinical acumen.

Preferred way is to through US guidance as its more accurate way of infiltrating PRP in the lesion. The intra-lesional PRP infiltration has distinct advantage than a wide spread non-specific infiltration.

1. Reparation of Autologous Fresh PRP through small volume venous blood about 3 ml.

2. Preparation of the site by using all aseptic precaution

3. Identification of the lesion/defect by USG.

4. Placing a needle in the lesion, under USG guidance and ensuring it is inside the lesion.

5. Infiltrate the PRP about 2–5ml in the lesion. Keep the USG Probe and Injection needle at Right angles for best visualization. (Figure No.54 A B C)

   At times this infiltration is very painful particularly in tennis elbow if penetrates the periosteum.

   Usually we prefer giving oral antibiotic coverage with single dose or for 3 days, if at high risk like diabetics.

6. The beneficial effects usually take s abut 5-21 days and are long lasting. (Figure 55)

7. The injections are repeated after 7and 21 days, particularly in recalcitrant and old lesions.

This is with the intention to stimulate the proliferative healing cycle.

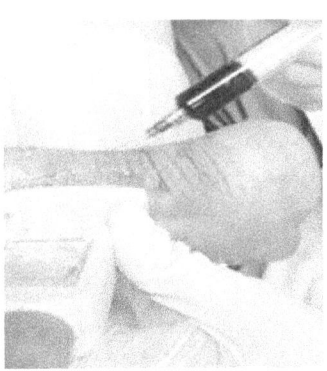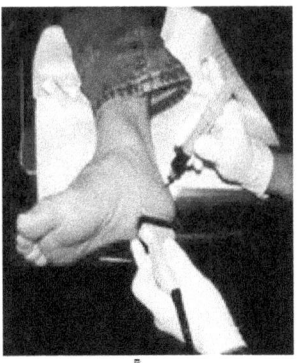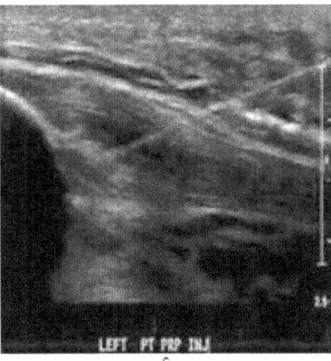

Figure 54: A: Showing placement of Needle and of USG Probe for Tendo-Achilitis

B. Showing placement of Needle & USG Probe for Plantar fascitis

C: USG guided Intra-lesional infiltration.

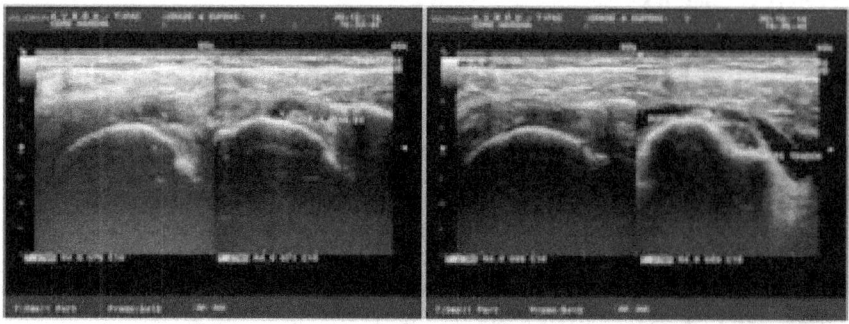

Pre infiltration ultrasonography revealed altered echoic pictures and thickening of tendon with associated bursitis and fluid collection around bursal surface of tendon. A tear observed on the bursal surface of the tendon . Grade III type of supraspinatus tear.

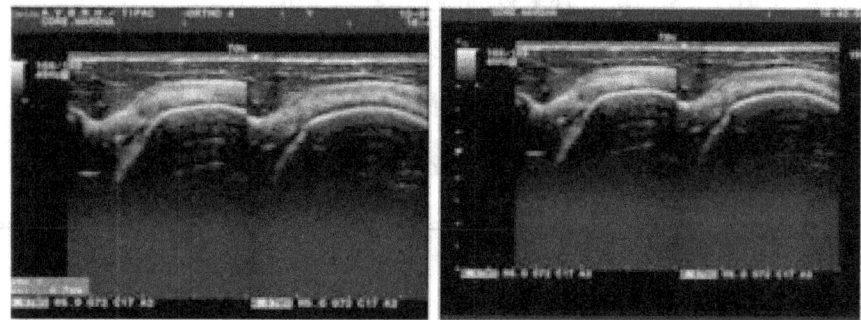

Follow up ultrasonography showed improved echoic pictures and thickening of tendon with associated mild bursitis. No fluid collection around bursal surface of tendon were noted.

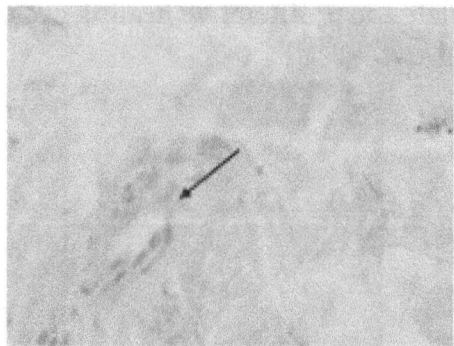

Histopatholaogy tendon biopsy – shows tenosynovial fibres with little disarraying with proliferating capillaries (neovascularization) suggesting repair phenomenon. (H & E, 40X)

Chapter V

PRP in Osteoarthritis of Knee

1

Introduction

Osteoarthritis is a degenerative disease, due to thinning and loss of elasticity of cartilages.

Many lines of treatments are available for different stages of this disease including both surgical and non-surgical interventions

The non-surgical are targeted towards knee joint preservation. These are mainly targeted towards control of pain and inflammation. Drugs including local intraarticular injection are used. The local injections include viscosupplementations by Hyaluronic acid infiltrations also to improve the dryness of joints. The other commonly used injections are of steroids.

The current attempts aimed at for cartilage- treatment; has been mainly towards Chondro-protection and includes drugs such as Cartilamine, Glucosamine etc.

With the "Regenerative Medicine" now being an intense treatment option available, the aim for cartilage –regeneration has to be included in the management line.

This inclusion of cartilage regeneration as an aim for treatment of OA knee is getting established.

The role of PRP is being investigated intensely and its clinical application in OA knee is now finding way as a part of regular treatment. But still the dose, duration and forms remain uncertain.

2

Rationale

The PRP with its rich source of Growth factors such as vascular endothelial growth factor (VEGF), platelet-derived growth factor (PDGF) and transforming growth factor-b (TGF-b) [1], alter the changing joint milieu in OA.

The PRP promotes the synthesis of Collagen II and prostaglandins through increasing the chondrocyte proliferation and strengthening of matrix.

The pathways for Chondrocyte apoptosis are influenced by IGF-1 downregulating the programmed cell death (PDCD5). This has a anabolic effects on both chondrocytes.

Similarly, influence of cytokines such as decreased IL-1, TNF alpha etc influences the synovial environment inside the joint and controls the inflammation.

Further the angiogenesis and formation of fibro-cartilaginous tissue should improve the cartilage thickness.

The pain control is also directly influenced at molecular (mRNA) levels leading to increae at CB1 And CB2 Cannabinoid) receptors.

All these are complex interactions are stimulated by the PRP infiltration, and are useful for triggering the Cartilage regenerations too.

Hence the PRP based therapy for OA knee offers additional advantages than other therapies by influencing all three aspects of OA – Inflammation, pain and Cartilage regeneration.

The metaanalysis by Robeh et al in 2016 concluded that PRP is clinically more effective the HA and Placebos.

A very useful review on various aspects of OA knee, has been published by Mandeep Dhillion et al in 2017.

3

Current Trends

Type of PRP:

The choice between leucocyte rich and Leucocyte poor PRP is still not so clear.

The different studies have demonstrated variability.

- 2012: Dragoo et al.: In rabbit model – that the Leucocyte rich group had more undesirable side effects owing to greater inflammatory reactions following injection at the lesion site than at the Leucocyte poor group

- 2012: Filardo et al.: Conducted a clinical trial comparing two different PRP preparations: high-concentrate leucocyte-rich PRP versus low concentrate leucocyte-free PRP. A comparable positive result was obtained in both treatments, with the PRP leucocyte group suffered from more swelling and pain reaction immediately after the injections.

- 2014- Pifer et al.: PRP with leucocytes contains MMP-2, –3 and –9, which is released over a period of at least six days, and can be deleterious.

- 2014 -Braun et al.: They compared the effects of leucocyte-rich PRP (LR-PRP), leucocyte-poor PRP (LP-PRP), red blood cell (RBC) concentrate and platelet-poor plasma (PPP) – "Treatment of synovial cells with LR-PRP and RBCs resulted in significant cell death and pro-inflammatory mediator production".

- 2014 Cavallo et al: Chondrocyte proliferation and hyaluronan secretion were more prevalent in L-PRP than in P-PRP

- 2016 Riboh et all: Conducted a meta-analysis and concluded that LP-PRP and LR-PRP had similar safety profiles, and adverse reactions to PRP may not be directly related to leucocyte concentration.

Overall it seems fresh autologous LP –PRP is a better option.

Dose and Duration

Still there is no clarity regarding PRP dosage and Scheduling's. Different researchers have tried differently. Dhillion et al reported that Single injection is as good as two injections; though recently multiple injection so PRP are reported to be a better option. The knee scores of Patients treated with 3 injections are found to be better. Mostly weekly or 3 week intervals have been advocated. But yearly use of PRP was also evaluated by Gobbi et al and clinical efficacy was established.

Approach:

There are two approaches by which the PRP can be infiltrated in the knee joint space.

Conventional suprapatellar injections or directly through anterior Para patellar approach.

Paterson et al in 2017 gave PRP intraosseous in the surrounding bones – femur, tibia and patella in addition to intraarticular.

PRP preparation

The PRP can be prepared by any method as described earlier.

The activated Platelets release 70% of Growth factors with 10 minutes and rest in 1 hour.

It should be noted that the controlled delivery of Growth Factors from PRP can be achieved by use of Scaffolds such as Chitsan and gelatin hydrogel. This has been demonstrated in animal models.

Synergistic effect with HA

Anitua et al, Marmotti et al and Andeia et al have propagated this concept that HA + PRP may be more useful than PRP alone. The results are controversial with Dalleri et al reporting no advantage and Lana et al reporting a better outcome.

Indications

The consensus is that Early OA knee is a good indication for PRP treatment.

Though few researchers (as mentioned above) have also propagated for late OA of knee.

In hip OA, recently arthroscopic assisted injections ar e propagated by Dalleri et al

4

Key Evidences in Literature

- 2008 Sánchez M, Anitua E, Azofra J, Aguirre JJ, Andia I: Established the safety of PRP for Intra-articular use.

- 2010: Kon et al: Gave 3 freeze thawed PRP injections at 3 weeks interval and noted improvement in IKDC and VAS scores.

- 2010 Engebretsen et al: The available clinical studies on PRP as a treatment option suggest a good potential in favoring pain reduction and improved function for articular injuries to the ankle, knee and hip

- 2011: Kon et al: 3 autologous fresh PRP injections at two weeks interval noted better and sustained results.

- 2011 Li et al: Better results in PRP than HA group at 6 months.

- 2012: Spakova et al: Demonstrated the safety profile and beneficial effects of PRP in early OA knee (grade 1,2,3 of Kellgren and Lawernce) with improvement in WOMAC score.

- 2012: Cerza et al: Gave 4 weekly PRP injections with better WOMAC scores in PRP group, independent of grade of OA.

- 2012: Snchez et al: 3 PPR at weekly interval were given. They noticed better outcomes in the PRP group at 24 weeks in respect to primary outcome as per 50% decrease in WOMAC pain scores. No differences for secondary outcome measures (WOMAC other sub scores, Lequesne index and OARSI) and amount of acetaminophen consumption were observed.

- 2013: Say et al: Better results with PRP than HA.

- 2013: Patel et al: Better results with PRP than Placebo (Normal Saline), at 6 months.

- 2014 Prieto-Alhambra et al: The effects of PRP seemingly last longer and are superior in comparison with intramuscular injection therapies.

- 2015 Kon et al: reported no superiority of PRP over Visco-supplementation

- 2017 Laver et al: PRP injections being considered a safe procedure with more favorable outcomes when compared to alternative treatments (

- 2018 Liam G Glynn et al: PRP therapy is a simple and minimally invasive intervention which is feasible to deliver in primary care to treat osteoarthritis. Improved outcomes were observed.

- 2018 Grassi et al.: In a meta-analysis, advocated PRP treatment as a safe procedure with negligible adverse effects that is readily available and has a minimal risk of reactivity compared to other exogenous compounds owing to the autologous nature of PRP injections.

- 2019 BrendanO'Connel et al: More uniformly positive results have been observed by various studies for PRP in OA knee in comparison to hyaluronic acid, other intra-articular injections and placebo than in o ther musculoskeletal tissue. Further research is required to investigate how leukocyte inclusion, activation and platelet concentration affect therapeutic efficacy. Furthermore, the optimisation of timing, dosage, volume, frequency and rehabilitation strategies need to be ascertained.

5

Our Experience

We conducted the study comparing PRP and local steroid infiltration.

The long-term effects of PRP are better, with improved WOMA scores and VAS scores.

Table 6,7 and Figure 56 & 57.

	PRP Group		Steroid Group		t-value	p-value
	Mean	SD	Mean	SD		
Baseline	59	13.55	58.36	12.47	0.24	0.80,NS
1 month	51.96	11.67	50.86	11.34	0.47	0.63,NS
3 months	48.08	10.69	55.64	11.56	3.39	0.001,S
6 months	43.62	10.33	61.68	12.48	7.99	0.0001,S

	PRP Group		Steroid Group		t-value	p-value
	Mean	SD	Mean	SD		
Baseline	6.26	1.00	6.50	1.07	1.15	0.25,NS
1 month	5.18	0.84	5.28	0.96	0.54	0.58,NS
3 months	4.66	0.74	5.92	1.12	6.61	0.0001,S
6 months	4.18	0.84	6.74	1.12	12.86	0.0001,S

Table 6: Comparison of WOMAC scores in PRP and Steroid groups using unpaired test

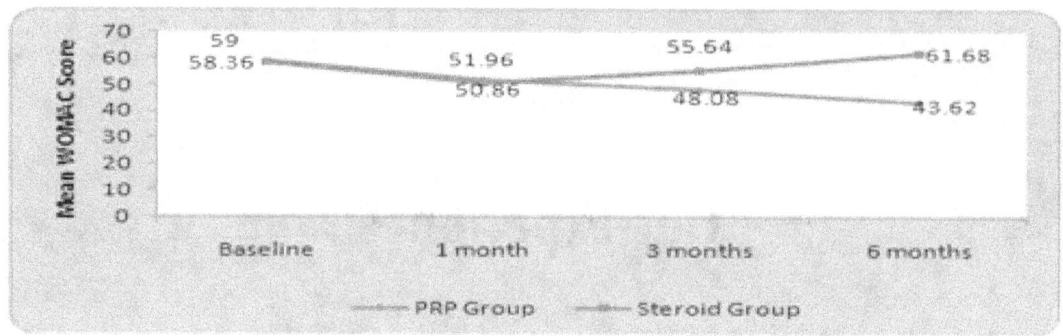

Figure 56: Graph comparing PRP and Steroid groups WOMAC score.

	PRP Group		Steroid Group		t-value	p-value
	Mean	SD	Mean	SD		
Baseline	6.26	1.00	6.50	1.07	1.15	0.25,NS
1 month	5.18	0.84	5.28	0.96	0.54	0.58,NS
3 months	4.66	0.74	5.92	1.12	6.61	0.0001,S
6 months	4.18	0.84	6.74	1.12	12.86	0.0001,S

Table 7: Showing Pain Comparison through VAS scores in PRP and Steroid Groups.

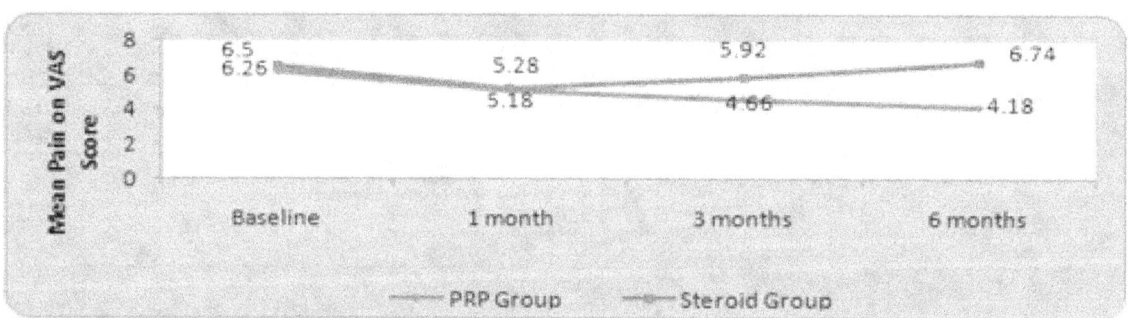

Figure57: Showing graph comparing the VAS scores in PRP and Steroid group.

Practice at our Centre

Indication:

- Early OA knee with no severe mechanical deformations and instabilities.
- Moderate OA with mild deformities.

Eligible Patients:

No blood dyscarisis/disorders and with normal platelet counts.

Technique:

1. Preparation: 3 ml of Fresh Autologous PRP (Leucocyte poor) prepared from double spin method with no activators from low volume venous blood.

2. The site is prepared with aseptic precautions as done for nay major interventional procedural.

3. Both approaches are used–

Suprapatellar and direct anterior direct (Figure number 18 and figure number 19).

The direct approach is used more now, particularly patients with inflamed synovium's.

Direct Anterior

- The knee is flexed to about 70-80 degrees.
- Joint line is palpated.
- Just superior to lateral tibial condyle the needle is inserted into the joint.
- It is ensured that needle do not pierce any structure and is freely moving inside the joint space.
- The needle used are of 20-22 G.
- About 3 ml of PRP is injected into the joint.
- The insertion site is sealed.
- Knee joint is gentle put through rage of movement to spread the fluid evenly.
- A compression bandage is applied; immediate full weight bearing is encouraged.

Usually after 4 hours the bandage is removed and ROM exercises stared.

Many Patients may have a mild exaggeration of pain and inflammation, which usually last for about 6–8 hours.

4. The Injections are usually repeated at 7 & 21 days. The rationale is stimulating the Proliferative stage of healing, as per the inflammatory cycle studies, which tend to start by 7 dyas and peak at 21 days.

5. In high risk cases, suitable Antibiotic is given for 3 days.

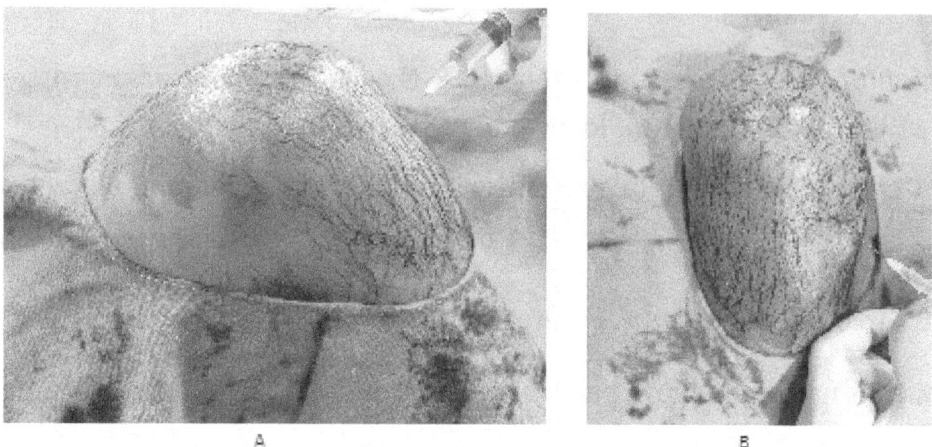

Figure 58: A: Anterior direct approach with knee in flexion

B: Anterior Direct approach just above the Lateral tibial condyle and Para -patellar.

Chapter VI

PRP for Fracture Impairments

1

Introduction

Fracture healing is a complicated metabolic process and requires the interaction of many factors, including the recruitment of reparative cells and genes. If these factors are inadequate or interrupted, healing is delayed or impaired, resulting in a non-union of the bone[. Complete fracture healing takes approximately 12 weeks to 24 months.

The bone healing process is a delicate balance between bone deposition, resorption, and remodelling. The fracture healing process undergo stages of: Hematoma formation, inflammation, formation of soft callus, formation of hard callus, and finally the bone remodeling process. (McKibbin,)

The current management requires the impaired healings to be intervened through Bone grafting procedures. Platelets provide exogenous source of growth factors stimulating the activity of bone cell's and are very exciting options towards treatment of fracture impairments.

2

Rationale

A. Role of Platelet Rich Plasma in Bone Healing

PRP serves as a growth factor agonist and has both mitogenic and chemotactic properties. It initiates repair by releasing locally acting growth factors via α-granules degranulation. The secretory proteins contained in the α-granules of platelets include platelet-derived growth factor (PDGF-AA, BB, and AB isomers), transforming growth factor-β (TGF-β), platelet factor 4 (PF4), interleukin-1 (IL-1), platelet-derived angiogenesis factor (PDAF), vascular endothelial growth factor (VEGF), epidermal growth factor (EGF), platelet-derived endothelial growth factor (PDEGF), epithelial cell growth factor (ECGF), insulin like growth factor (IGF), osteocalcin (Oc), osteonectin (On), fibrinogen (Ff), vitronectin (Vn), fibronectin (Fn) and thrombospondin-1 (TSP-1). Platelets are the richest source of TGF-β, having both isoform TGF-β1 and TGF-β2 in it. TGF-β1 has the greatest potential for bone repair, and TGF-β may contribute to bone healing at all stages. The PDGF and TGF-β1 promote the proliferation and differentiation of osteoblasts while TGF-β1 also has the ability to inhibit the differentiation of adipocyte. PRP is osteoinductive for impairment of the bone healing process. The platelets in PRP are further activated by bone substitution materials and biphasic osteochondral scaffolds.

B. Role of Platelet Rich Plasma in Osteoporotic Fracture Healing

The osteoporotic bones present a difficult challenge due to poor bone quality. The treatments are aimed to preserve bone mass, and decrease fracture risk. In case of fracture of such bones, application of growth factors and systemic administration of agents promoting bone formation can be the better treatment option. As per Lopez et al in 2003, the healing of osteoporotic bone is slow in progress and takes a longer period, otherwise its same as in any other fractures. But now there are evidences of altered fracture healing in osteoporotic bone There are few evidence published regarding the role of

PRP in osteoporotic fractures in special relation with different growth factors (TGF, FGF, VEGF, EGF, etc.) secreted by platelets. The optimum concentration of growth factors at fracture site, enhances the rate of progression of healing and improves the quality of new bone formation. Liu *et al.* showed the therapeutic role of PRP in osteoporosis with the evidence that the PRP not only inhibit the maturation of preadipocytes (3T3-L1) into adipocyte but also promotes osteogenesis. As per Muruganandan *et al.* PRP-induced osteogenesis in osteoporotic fractures is achieved by simultaneously up-regulating osteogenesis-promoting genes Runx2, OPN, and OCN while downregulating adipogenesis regulators such as PPAR-g2 and leptin. The PRP treatment also enhanced BMP-2 and BMP receptor type IB (BMPR-IB) and suppressed BMPR-IA pathways in preadipocytes. In addition to these studies, more researchers observed the same and concluded that the transdifferentiation of adipocytes to osteoblasts was possible without genetic manipulation.

3

Key Evidence in Literature

- 2005: Okuda K et al: Treatment with a combination of PRP and Hydroxyapatite compared to Hydroxyapatite with saline led to a significantly more favorable clinical improvement in intrabony periodontal defects.

- 2005: Coetzee JC et al: Agility total ankle replacements were performed without and with autologous concentrated growth factors for distal syndesmosis fusion the result of which was that autologous concentrated growth factors appeared to make a significant positive difference in the syndesmosis union rate in total ankle replacements.

- 2008: Galsso et al: Used a combination of self-locking intramedullary nailing and PRP for treatment of atrophic diaphyseal long bone non-unions and reported a healing rate of 91%. They did not apply autologous bone grafting.

- 2010: Hakimi et al: PRP along with autologous grafts in animal model, reported significantly better regeneration

- 2010: Huang S et al: Optium concentration of PRP improves the osteogenesis and osteoinduction.

- 2011 Kanthan Sr et al: PRP in combination with bone grafting improved the bone healing rate of rabbit when compared to bone graft alone. They also demonstrated that use of PRP alone (without bone grafting) does not affect the outcome and healing rate and provides limited advantage over placebo.

- 2011: Hakimi et al: In a clinical study reported the successful treatment of 17 patients with persistent non-union of long bones using combination of PRP and autologous bone grafting

- 2014: Say et al: Did not observed adequate healing in nonunion with PRP alone.

- 2014: Lee et al: Used autologous bone marrow aspirate concentrate combined with PRP injection at the osteotomy site. It helped improve bone healing in distraction osteogenesis of the tibia.

- 2015: Malhotra et al: PRP for nonunion of long bones had good results

- 2016: Fairborz et al: Found that healing was significantly higher in PRP group as compared to placebo group in the population of Long bones fracture treated additionally with PRP, along with Nail and grafts. It was also associated with lower pain scores. Application of PRP along with autologous bone graft in the site of non-union of long bone after intramedullary nailing or ORIF results in higher cure rate, shorter healing duration, lower limb shortening and less postoperative pain. Higher infection rate might be a complication of PRP application

The evidence points to following interesting aspects of PRP for its application in fracture impairment:

- It is more beneficial to use in early healing phase than later.

- It is more useful to use in association with some scaffolds such as autologous bone grafts or distraction osteogenesis.

- The osteoinduction and osteogenesis is concentration dependent and a medium concentration of ($2.5 - 4.5 \times 10^9$) is most suitable. A very high concentration and very low concentration of PRP show no capability in the osteoinductive stimulations.

- The PRP effects the healing in the osteoporotic bones too.

4

Our Experience

We had been using PRP alone, mainly

- For inducing union in infective non-unions (Figure 59A, B, C)
- Very interestingly we have also used it for treatment of infective diaphysis of bone with potential fracture. (Figure 60 A, B, C) for consolidation of involucrum ; and
- Consolidation of regenerate after distraction osteogenesis. (Figure 61 AB).

  In such cases the PRP infiltration is started a on achieving the desired bone lengthening., to avoid any premature consolidation.

The infiltrations are done on 0, 7, 21 days and were repeated after every 3 weeks in recalcitrant non-union, after radiological reviews.

Repeated PRP infiltrations at fracture site have resulted in a good union.

A key observation in such cases is that once the PRP infiltration was undertaken as intervention in towards consolidating the regenerate, the time to consolidate become stable at around 8-10 weeks, independent of the length of regenerate.

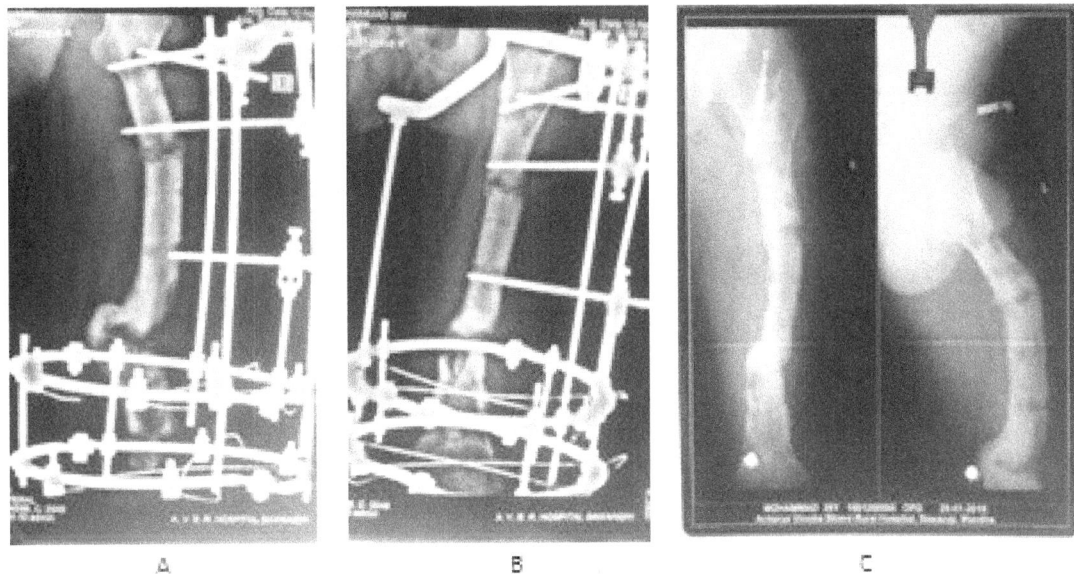

Figure 59: A & B: Xrays showing infected Non union at Distal Femur sites & Poor Regnerate at Proximal femur site.

C: After PRP treatment at both sites – Union is achived. Post PRP radiological pictures in Infected nonunion.

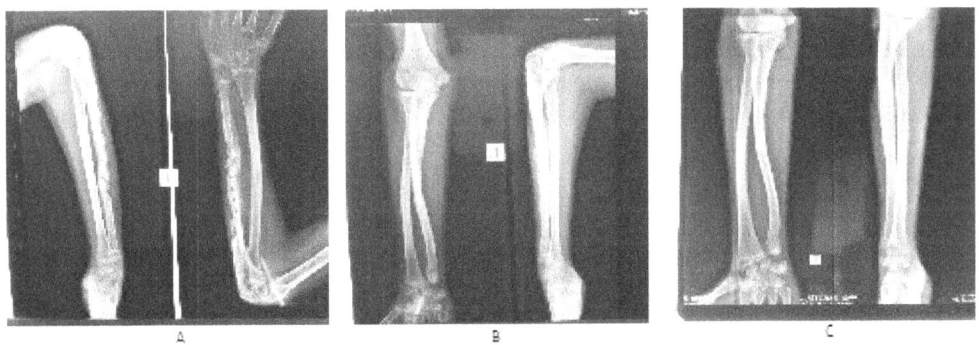

Figure 60: A: Xray -AP & Lat. View showing Chronic Osteomyelitis of Ulna

B: Xray – AP & Lat. View showing Involucrum consolidation with PRP treatment

C: Xray – AP & Lat. View showing consolidation of involucrum in chronic osteomyelitis with absorption of Sequestrum after two of completion of treatment.

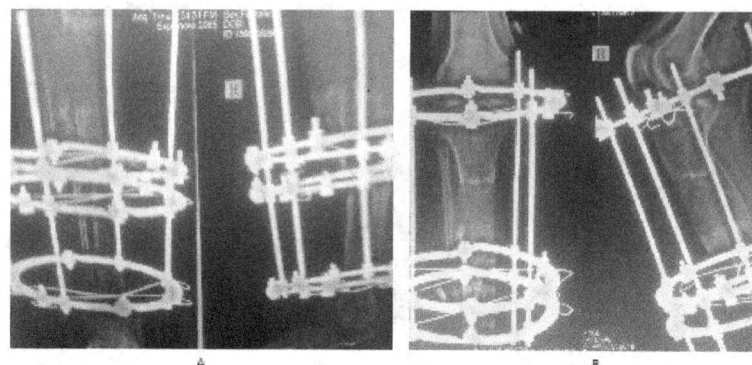

Figure 61: A: Xray AP & Lat. Views showing poor regenerate after lengthening
B: Xray AP & Lat. Views showing consolidation of Regenerate after PRP infiltration

Steps for PRP Infiltration

Indications:

- Fractures showing a small distraction/ gaps after implant fixations
- Fractures going into delayed unions
- Non-unions along with stabilization procedures, including infective non-union.
- Consolidations of poor involucrum in Chromic osteomyelitis
- Consolidation of regenerate after distraction osteogenesis.

Eligible Patients:

- Patient with no blood dyscarisis / disorders and normal platelet counts.
- Haemoglobin of atleast 10 gm% as repeated infiltrations are done.

Technique:

Figure 62 A B C

- All procedures are performed under IITV –C ARM.
- PRP is prepared by standard methods from low volume (20-50ml autologous venous blood)
  o Usually no activation process is now being used.
- The site is identified under C-ARM.
- All aseptic precautions are undertaken as per major interventional procedure.
- Local anaesthesia is given at the site from which penetration of a wide bore needle is planned.
- A Needle of 18 G is usually used.

- o Many times, spinal needles are used for extra length to reach at the site of non-union.

- 3-5 ml of PRP is injected in the non-union site.

The injection is repeated on 7tth day and then on 21st day. After that radiological monitoring is done on every 21st day and PRP continued till union is seen or up to 12 weeks, whichever is early.

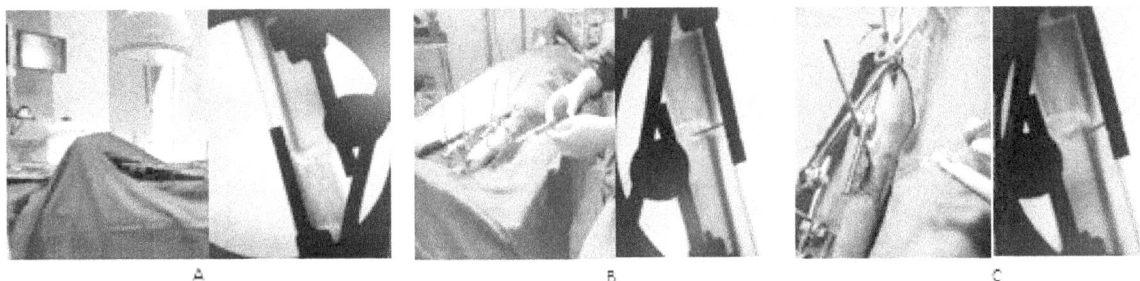

Figure 62: A. Identification of fracture site under C-arm-IITV

B. Infiltration of PRP inside the Nonunion

C. Infiltration in surrounding area.

Chapter VII

PRP in Subfertility/ Infertility.

1

Endometrium Regeneration

A. Introduction:

Success of any IVF cycle depends on favourable interaction between healthy embryos and adequately thick, responsive endometrium.

Adequate endometrial thickness is a main factor for implantation and pregnancy. Women with persistent thin endometrium often cancelled to undergo embryo transfer

The optimum thickness of endometrium for conducive implantation environment should be is , a matter debate .

Different sets of thickness are said to minimally present for better outcomes. These are

- ≥6 mm: Gonenet al, 1990; Shapiro et al, 1993; Coulamet al, 1994
- 7 mm: Rinaldiet al, 1996;Kovacs et al 2003; Zhang et al, 2005; Richter et al, 2007; El-Toukhyet al, 2008; Kumbaket al, 2009.
- >8mm: Gingoldet al, 2015

The may be controversies in exact thickness but what is certain is t.his is the "Rate – Limiting step" in reproduction. Refractory thin endometrium plays a significant part in its receptivity

The thin refractory endometrium is managed with lots of variations & uncertainties. The quest for health endometrium have evolved many solutions including:

- Exogenous estrogen,
- Low- dose aspirin,
- Vitamin E
- Vaginal sildenafil citrate·

- Pentoxyphyline ,
- L-arginine,
- Electroacupuncture,

With regenerative medicine , yielding biological solutions for regeneration, the Growth factors and Stem cells are also being used for the same, including:

- Application of granulocyte colony stimulation factor (G-CSF),
- Intrauterine infusion of bone marrow mesenchymal cells,
- Autologous adult stem cells, and
- Autologous Platelet rich plasma.

The Use of PRP has distinct advantages as has been outlined in chapter of Basics of PRP.

B. Key Evidences

Local infusion of PRP that contains several growth factors and cytokines may improve endometrial growth and receptivity.

For the first time, Chang reported the efficacy of intrauterine infusion of PRP for endometrial growth in women with thin endometrium. In that trial, PRP was infused in 5 women with inadequate endometrium who had poor response to conventional therapy during the FET cycle. The proper response to treatment was reported in all of them, and normal pregnancy was reported in 4 women.

The Shahrzad Zadehmodarres, et al, PRP has been considered as a safe procedure, with minimal risks of transmission of infectious disease and immunological reactions since it is made from autologous blood samples. Adequate endometrial growth was found in all the participants after two PRP infusions in all patients who had a history of cycle cancellation due to thin endometrium

C. Our Experience

Eligible Patients: Infertility with thin endometrium (≤ 7 mm), on the day of hCG administratio

Inclusion criteria

- Age: 30–45 years.
- Previous cycle cancellations due to of thin unresponsive endometrium, in spite of treatment.
- Normal uterine cavity (Confirmed by Hysteroscopy).

Exclusion criteria

o   Presence of systemic diseases, endocrine disorders, sickle cell disease, chronic neutropenia, history of malignancy and renal insufficiency.

o   Women with Haemoglobin < 10 g/dl , Platelet count < 1lac per microliter

o   Presence of Asherman's syndrome, fibroids, and polyps on hysteroscopy.

Technique:

1.   Autologous PRP was prepared under all aseptic precautions from 7.5ml of autologous venous blood in 2.5ml of citrate solution, by double spin method at room temperature. (Figure ABC & Figure ABC).

2.   0.5 to 1.5 ml of PRP yield was obtained.

3.   1st Infusion was done into the uterine cavity with Intrauterine Catheter on 10th day of hormone replacement therapy of frozen embryo transfer

4.   The Endometrial thickness was re-assed after 48 - 72 hours.

5.   Second infusion was given if Endometrium failed to grow more than 7mm.

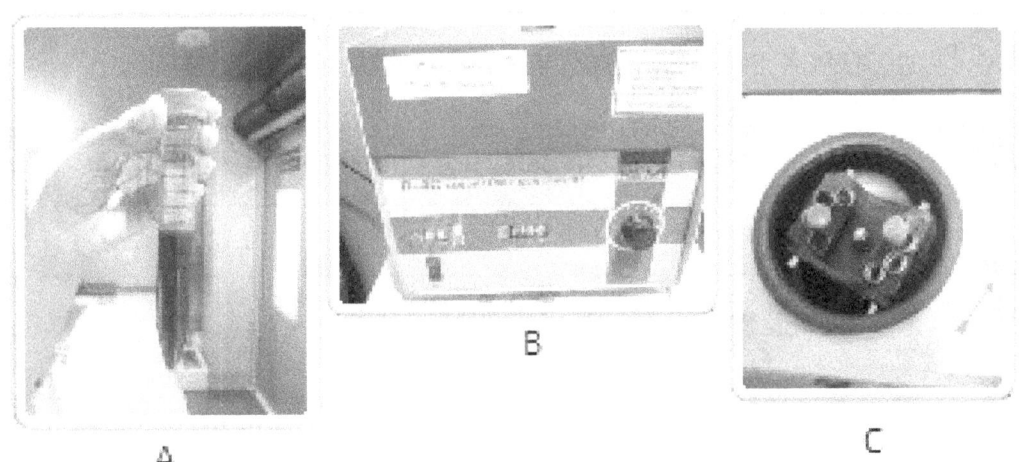

Figure 63: I Spin

Figure 63: A. Collection for 7.5 ml of blood

B. Centrifuge 1200rpm x 10min

C. Counter balancing inside machine.

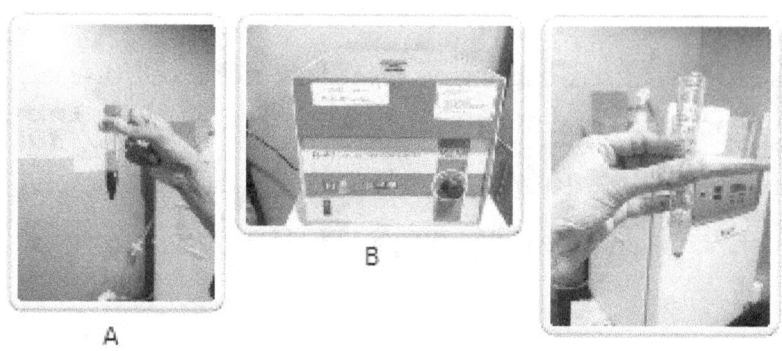

Figure 64: II Spin

Figure 64: A. Separation in 3 layers

B. Centrifuge 2000rpm x 10min

C. The PRP with pelle.

Out come assessment: Through serial ultrasound & Doppler, after evry 2 days; prior to embryo transfer date, measuring the increase in endometrial thickness and vascularity.

Significant increase of endometrial thickness (ET) and improvement in endometrial vascularity (measured as per Apllebaum zonal scoring) in zone I to zone IV.

The results of 10 Patients are as per Table 8 & 9 and Figure 65

Figure	PRE-INFUSION ET	POST INFUSIONET	IMPROVEMENT INET	P value
PRP	5.96 ± 0.58	7.18 ± 0.84	1.22	<0.01

Table 8: Showing Gain in Endometrial thickness

	PRE-INFUSION VASCULARITY	POST INFUSION VASCULARITY	IMPROVEMENT IN VASCULARITY	P value
PRP	2.16 ± 0.80	3.68 ± 0.23	1.52	<0.01

Table 9: Showing Improvement in Vascularity

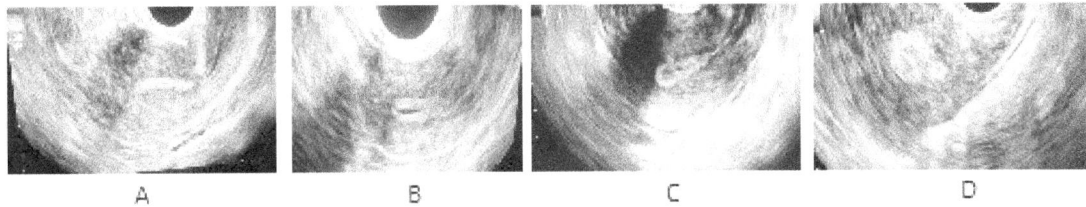

Figure 65: Serial USG for Endometrium Regeneration

A. The thin Endometrium

B. PRP instillation in ET (Fluid seen inside Endometrium)

C. After 2 days – Endometrium seen thickening

D. Final Endometrial regeneration with adequate thick endometrium.

Other Parameters

The PRP was found to be safe with no major adverse events observed (Table10)

SN	PARAMETERS	
1	Pain & tenderness	1
2	Bleeding	Nil
3	Fluid collection in endometrium	Nil
4	Infection	Nil
5	Erythematous skin lesion	Nil

Table 10: Showing any untoward effect after PRP infusion in endometrium.

2

Ovarian Rejuvenation

Improving Ovarian Reserve Amongst Women with Low AMH

A. Introduction:

PRP has been an "ovarian rejuvenation treatment" to help women overcome premature menopause, low ovarian reserves, and advanced maternal age.

The same way PRP stimulates tissue growth in injured athletes, it can stimulate oocyte production in a woman's ovaries.

Being a newer modality of treatment not much is published in literature.

The few important evidences are as following:

- E. Scott Sills et al. have reported that direct injection of activated PRP into the human ovary of poor prognosis IVF patients. Evidence of improved ovarian function was noted in all who received intraovarian PRP, possibly as early as two months after treatment

- Aleksandra Ljubić et al have reported the possibilities of genetic treatment of the ovarian tissue in order to restore both reproductive and endocrine functions of the ovary. This is perhaps the first case of human embryo obtained after autologous PRP in vitro activation of ovaries by interrupting PRP stimulating AKT pathway with ultrasound-guided orthotropic re-transplantation.

- Pantos K et have reported for the first time, the successful temporary ovarian activity restoration in perimenopausal women after an autologous ovarian platelet-rich plasma treatment.

B. Our Experience:

We have conducted the procedure at our IVF Centre, with aim to observe the role of PRP for increasing ovarian reserve in women of low AMH seeking treatment of infertility at AVBRH.

The study is conducted on 12 Women, having poor ovarian reserve.

Eligibility

Inclusion Criteria.

1. Woman whose previous cycles were anovulatory in USG guided follicular study.

2. Woman between 20 to 45 years of age group with low AMH.

3. Woman in whom previous IVF cycles could not provide good oocyte yield even after adequate stimulation

Exclusion Criteria

1. Family or past history of cancer,

2. Hb<10 g/dL, platelets <150,000/mm3,

3. NSAIDs in the 10 days before procedure

4. Any significant comorbidity or psychiatric disorder that would compromise patient safety or compliance, interfere with consent, study participation, follow up, or interpretation of study results.

5. Incision in the uterus: myomectomy; caesarean section.

6. 7-Any active infection or illness.

Technique:

- Diagnostic Hysterolaproscopy is performed in the pretreatment cycle.

- PRP preparation with double spin method, from 10 ml autologous venous blood, as shown in Figures

- PRP instillation was performed Laparoscopic guidance, in the same sitting.
  - o USG guidance was noted in whom Previous laparoscopic opportunity for PRP instillation was missed.

- The routine protocol is followed:-

- Day 21 –Long Agonist protocol with Leuoprolide 0.5mg/l/sc till the day of stimulation in next cycle.

- Ovarian stimulation For Day 2 of menses 300 HMG /IM and 0.3 mg /l/sc leuoprolide was given subcutaneous, till 6th day. Follicular scan done. The dose of gonadotropins is individualized according to the patient's age and previous stimulation history or response to stimulation.

- Cycles will be monitored by Trans Vaginal Ultrasonography and serum Estradiol, FSH, LH and Progesterone levels.

- Follicular maturation is completed by the administration of 10,000 IU hCG injection or injection leuprolide 0.2mg, when at least two follicles have reached a diameter of >17 mm. After embryo-transfer luteal support is carried out by using 100 mg/day of progesterone injection.

Results analysis:

- Good quality embryos are defined as four cells on Day 2 or 8 or more cells on Day 3, grade 1–2 defined as embryos with 0–20% of fragmentation.

- Positive pregnancy is defined as a β-hCG level>100mIU/mL, 14Days following embryo-transfer, and

- Clinical pregnancy is identified by the appearance of a gestational sac approximately 4 weeks after embryo replacement.

PRP could be used as a first line treatment for the ovarian regeneration and the folliculogenesis reactivation of peri-menopausal women. PRP therapy may extend the fertility potential of peri-menopausal women, rendering oocyte donation IVF cycle as an ultimatum option.

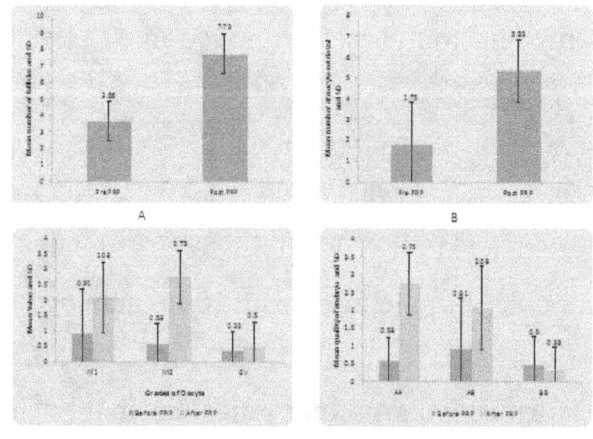

Figure 65: A: Comparison of number of follicle before and after PRP

B: Comparison of number of oocyte retrieval before and after PRP

C: Comparison of grades of oocyte before and after PRP

D: Comparison of quality of embryo before and after PRP

The PRP triggered regeneration can help in improving the outcomes of Sub fertility treatments by stimulating the regenerations at the

Endometrium and Ovary.

Summary & Conclusion

The Regenerative Medicine is changing the way the diseases are & will be treated.

It brings a lot of optimism with newer options, after centuries of development of Surgical and Pharmaceutical interventions.

The PRP are the simplest Regenerative Medicine product, which is currently available for the clinical applications.

Its use in Musculoskeletal disorders, Wounds and Infertility management is bring huge hope for millions.

It is lowering the morbidity and improving the prognosis for many complex health problems.

More importantly, newer solutions are getting successfully implemented, for hereto hopeless situations, as seen in cases of gangrenes. The days are not far away, when mortality will also be under control with these interventions.

Development of STARS therapy is a small step towards standardization of the current practices.

But a big leap in for management of complex wounds, overcoming many challenges.

It is just an indication, for what is in store in the future for health care.

The 21st century will see the regenerating medicine competing with technology for dominance, which is good news for whole human kind. This, if goes in symbiotic manner, will break many barriers and lead health towards predictable and better care.

We hope that this attempt to give an insight & preparedness to handle PRP will be fruitful, to all our readers.

List of Figures & Tables

FigureNo.	Detail
1	Different PRP preparations and the Growth factors.
2	Role Different Growth Factors during Tissue regeneration
3	Blood Fractionation: Cells, whole blood, plasma
4	PRP Method
5	A typical commercial kit for PRP Preparation
6	A Pre- programmed centrifuge Machines.
7	Showing Blood being withdrawn from antecubital vein
8 A	Transfer of equal quantity of blood in 4 bulbs.
8 B	Placement in the centrifuge machine loading with counter balancing
9	Separation of blood into Buffy coat and RBC layer.
10	Further separation into u ½ of mainly WBC and Lower PRP
11A	Margin Preparation with Povidone iodine
11 B	Further cleaning with Alcohol and normal saline
12	Swab Collection for Culture & Sensitivity
13A	Side way to infiltrate PRP in regenerating skin margins
13B	Direct way to infiltrate PRP in regenerating skin margins
13C	From normal skin way to infiltrate PRP in regenerating skin margins
14	Do not infiltrate in wound
15	Infiltrations into the progressive regenerating skin margins
16A	Peaking of Proliferative Phase on day 4th, during wound healing.
16B	Correlation between CRP- value and days.

FigureNo.	Detail
17	Report bacterial cultures in PRP and bacterial growths in it.
18A, B, C, D	Serial Photographs of foot showing cicterization
19A	Infected postoperative wound -MRSA positive
19B	Complete healing of Infected MRSA positive post caesarean w ound.
20A	Pouring pus in compound fracture – MRSA positive
20B	After 4 sessions: Complete infection Control
20C	After 8 sessions: Complete healing
21A	Progressive postoperative flap necrosis with infection
21B	After 2 sessions: Showing the damage restriction & limited to dry small superficial necrotic patch
22A	Dirty wound with necrotizing bone & tendon
22B	After 2 sessions: Angiogenesis in both bone & tendon
22C	After 4 sessions: Coverage by healthy granulation tissue
23A	Showing Trophical Ulcer over foot.
23B	Complete healing.
23C	Recurrence after 4 months and a new ulcer after faulty Foot wear usage.
24A	Showing exposed Muscles of Leg & Tibia bone: Developing necrosis.
24B	The Stage of Suppression of Unhealthy tissue: Showing the appearance of speckles of angiogenesis in muscles and bone.
25 A	Infected chronic non-healing diabetic Ulcer
25B	Stage of Suppression of unhealthy Tissue
25C	Stage of Healthy Granulation
25D	Stage of Defect-filling
25E	Stage of Maturation of Epithelization
26A	After 48 hours: Phagocytic infiltration
26B	After 10 days: Defect filling with Angiotic tissue
26C	After 21 days: Complete filling up of defect with collagen tissue
26D	After 6 Weeks: Full thickness matured collagen led complete healing
27	Illustrative Case: 4 years old child, run over injury leading to partial loss of lateral aspect of foot
28	Illustrative Case: 33 years old Man sustained wound in road traffic accident – Compound fracture with exposed cut tendons with loss of skin.
29	Foot Reconstruction: 28 year old man sustained injury after road traffic accident , leading to Mangled extremity with loss of 4 metatarsal and 5 phalanges
30	A Mangled distal foot with all bones exposed and severe tissue loss

FigureNo.	Detail
31	22 years Male: Developed gas gangrene after injury of leg and foot
32	38 years male: upper limb injury, a deep wound with infection extending across the elbow
33	28 years old male: compound fracture of tibia with exposed bone and tendon.
34	55 years old Female:7 years old Venous ulcer over lateral aspect of lower leg and ankle.
35	22 years female – 5 years old Non-healing ulcer with juvenile diabetes & uncontrolled Sugar level.
36	72 years Male: Non- healing with Chronic osteomyelitis of Calcaeneum with diabetes.
37	65 years female: Bed sore, following prolonged immobilization due to Polytrauma, with diabetes
38	45 years male: Infected Pressure sore over skull after prolong Coma.
39	65 years old female with diabetes – Non-healing Wound after spinal decompression.
40	42 years old female – Wound dehiscence after Hysterectomy.
41	27 years old male - Postoperative following skin flap necrosis exposing the underneath implants.
42	29 years female: After Giant Cell Tumor removal of distal radius - Flap necrosis
43	18 years old girl: Developing gangrene of toes and flap necrosis, after sustaining injury in road traffic accident.
44	62 years Male: Severe infection of hand with gangrenous changes in all fingers, with Uncontrolled Diabetes.
45	15 years boy – Compound type III C (Gustilo & Anderson) fracture with bone loss of tibia
46	52 years Male: Gangrene of leg following compartment syndrome.
47	57 years Female: 2 days old road traffic injury with loss of skin and soft tissues with vascular deficit.
48	Clnacy's Classification for Tendinopathy
49	The Cellular phase of Tendon healing
50	A: Left forefoot at 3 weeks – Inflammatory Response B: Left forefoot at 12 weeks – Inflammatory Cells and Granulation tissue C: Left hind foot at 3 Weeks: Sparse Inflammatory cells and Fibrous Tissue D: left Hind foot at 12 weeks: Inflammatory infiltrate granulation tissue with Fibrous tissue
51	A: Right forefoot at 3 weeks: Inflammatory infiltrate and granulation tissue with Myocytes regeneration B: Right forefoot at 12 weeks: Fibro-collagenase tissue. C: Right Hind foot at 3 weeks: Fibro-collagenase tissue D: Right Hind foot: Fibro –collagenase tissue

FigureNo.	Detail
52	A. Left Fore foot – Primary repair. B. Left Hind foot – Defect 10mm C: PRP induced healings in primary repair. D: PRP induced healing in Gap.
53	A. Grade I lesion: FANC after 7 months of PRP infiltration: Tendon fibres with reacting tenosynovial cell activity along with fibro-collagenous material B: Grade II lesion: FNAC after 8 months of PRP infiltration tendon fibres with reactive fibrocytes and Fibro-collagenous tissue
54	A: Showing placement of Needle and of USG Probe for Tendo-Achilitis B. Showing placement of Needle & USG Probe for Plantar fascitis C: USG guided Intra-lesional infiltration.
55	Grade III lesions – USG and Histological pictures after PRP infiltration.
56	Graph comparing PRP and Steroid groups WOMAC score.
57	Figure57: Showing graph comparing the VAS scores in PRP and Steroid group.
58	A: Anterior direct approach with knee in flexion B: Anterior Direct approach just above the Lateral tibial condyle and Para –patellar.
59	A & B: Xrays showing infected Non union at Distal Femur sites & Poor Regnerate at Proximal femur site. C: After PRP treatment at both sites – Union is achived
60	A: Xray -AP & Lat. View showing Chronic Osteomyelitis of Ulna B: Xray – AP & Lat. View showing Involucrum consolidation with PRP treatment C: Xray – AP & Lat. View showing consolidation of involucrum in chronic osteomyelitis with absorption of Sequestrum after two of completion of treatment.
61	A: Xray AP & Lat. Views showing poor regenerate after lengthening B: Xray AP & Lat. Views showing consolidation of Regenerate after PRP infiltration.
62	A. Identification of fracture site under C-arm-IITV. B. Infiltration of PRP inside the Nonunion. C. Infiltration in surrounding area.
63	A. Collection for 7.5 ml of blood B. Centrifuge 1200rpm x 10min C. Counter balancing inside machine

FigureNo.	Detail
64	A. Separation in 3 layers
	B. Centrifuge 2000rpm x 10min
	C. The PRP with pellet.
65	A. The thin Endometrium
	B. PRP instillation in ET (Fluid seen inside Endometrium)
	C. After 2 days – Endometrium seen thickening
	D. Final Endometrial regeneration with adequate thick endometrium.

Table No.	Detail
1	Showing different growth factors and their primary role2
2	Effect of Growth Factors on Microenvironment during tissue regeneration
3	Platelet count and achieved by different authors at variable centrifuge speeds and time.
4	Showing day-wise changes during tendon repair
5	Showing the Evidence of Tendon healing by PRP in Rabbit
6	Comparison of WOMAC scores in PRP and Steroid groups using unpaired test
7	Showing Pain Comparison through VAS scores in PRP and Steroid Groups.
8	Showing Gain in Endometrial thickness
9	Showing Improvement in Vascularity
10	Showing any untoward effect after PRP infusion in endometrium

Acknowledgements and Reference for Further Reading

PRP - Properties and Preparations

- Blajchman MA Novel platelet products, substitutes and alternatives. Transfus Clin Biol 2001: 8, 267–271

- Tang YQ, Yeaman MR, Selsted ME Antimicrobial peptides from human platelets. Infect Immun 2002: 70: 6524-6533.

- Marx RE (Platelet-rich plasma: evidence to support its use. J Oral Maxillofac Surg 2004: 62: 489-496.

- De Somer F, De Brauwer V, Vandekerckhove M, Ducatelle R, Uyttendaele D, Van Nooten G. Can autologous thrombin with a rest fraction of ethanol be used safely for activation of concentrated autologous platelets applied on nerves? Eur Spine J 2006; 15:501-5.

- Everts PA, Brown Mahoney C, Hoffmann JJ, et al. Platelet-rich plasma preparation using three devices: implications for platelet activation and platelet growth factor release. Growth Factors. 2006; 24: 165-71

- Anitua E, Sanchez M, Orive G, et al. The potential impact of the preparation rich in growth factors (PRGF) in different medical fields. Biomaterials 2007: 28, 4551–4560.

- Bielecki TM, Gazdzik TS, Arendt J, Szczepanski T, Król W, et al. Antibacterial effect of autologous platelet gel enriched with growth factors and other active substances: An in vitro study. J Bone Joint Surg Br 2007: 89: 417-420.

- Mehta S, Watson JT. Platelet rich concentrate: basic science and current clinical applications. J Orthop Trauma. 2008; 22(6):432–8.

- Singh RP, Marwaha N, Malhotra P, Dash S. Quality assessment of platelet concentrates prepared by platelet rich plasma platelet concentrate, buffy coat poor platelet concentrates (BCPC) and apheresis PC methods. Asian J Transfus Sci. 2009; 3:86–94.

- Arora NS, Ramanayake T, Ren YF, Romanos GE. Platelet-rich plasma: A literature review. Implant Dent 2009; 18:303-10.

- Dohan Ehrenfest DM, Bielecki T, Del Corso M, Inchingolo F, Sammartino G. Shedding light in the controversial terminology for platelet-rich products: Platelet-rich plasma (PRP), platelet-rich fibrin (PRF), platelet-leukocyte gel (PLG), preparation rich in growth factors (PRGF), classification and commercialism. J Biomed Mater Res A 2010; 95:1280-2.

- Arnoczky SP, Delos D, Rodeo SA What is platelet-rich plasma? Oper Tech Sports Med 2011; 19(3), 142–148.

- Mazzocca AD, McCarthy MBR, Chowaniec DM, et al. Platelet-rich plasma differs according to preparation method and human variability. J Bone Joint Surg (Am) 2012 94(4), 308–316.

- Sánchez-González DJ, Méndez-Bolaina E, Trejo-Bahena NI Platelet rich plasma peptides: Key for regeneration. Int J Pept 2012: 532519.

- Boswell SG, Cole BJ, Sundman EA, et al. Platelet-rich plasma: a milieu of bioactive factors. Arthroscopy 2012; 28(3), 429–439.

- Busilacchi A, Gigante A, Mattioli-Belmonte M, et al. Chitosan stabilizes platelet growth factors and modulates stem cell differentiation toward tissue regeneration. Carbohydr Polym 2013; 98(1), 665–676

- Pifer MA, Maerz T, Baker KC, et al. Matrix metalloproteinase content and activity in low-platelet, low-leukocyte and high-platelet, high-leukocyte platelet rich plasma (PRP) and the biologic response to PRP by human ligament fibroblasts. Am J Sports Med 2014; 42(5), 1211–1218.

- Landesberg R, Moses M, Karpatkin M. Risks of using platelet rich plasma gel. J Oral Maxillofac Surg

PRP & Wounds

- Liu Y, Kalén A, Risto O, Wahlström O. Fibroblast proliferation due to exposure to a platelet concentrate in vitro is pH dependent. Wound Repair Regen 2002; 10:336-40.

- Eppley BL, Woodell JE, Higgins J. Platelet quantification and growth factor analysis from platelet-rich plasma: implications for wound healing. Plast Reconstr Surg. 2004;114(6):1502–8.

- McAleer JP, Sharma S, Kaplan EM, Persich G Use of autologous platelet concentrate in a nonhealing lower extremity wound. Adv Skin Wound Care 2006 19: 354-363.

- Pietramaggiori G, Kaipainen A, Czeczuga JM, Wagner CT, Orgill DP Freeze-dried platelet-rich plasma shows beneficial healing properties in chronic wounds. Wound Repair Regen 2006 14: 573-580.

- Greer N, Foman N, Dorrian J, et al. Advanced wound care therapies for non-healing diabetic, venous, and arterial ulcers: a systematic review. 2012.

- Martinez-Zapata MJ, Martí-Carvajal AJ, Solà I, et al. Autologous platelet rich plasma for treating chronic wounds. Cochrane Database Syst Rev. Issue 10 ,2012;

- Sandeep Shrivastava, Pradeep K. Singh, Shounak Taywade . STARS therapy: Sandeep's technique for assisted regeneration of skin. Journal of Orthopedics and Allied Sciences 2016; 4 (1):5-7.

- Shrivastava S, Mahakalkar C, Tayde S, Mehmood M, Gupta A Developing Ideal Solution for Acute Wound Treatment by Regenerative Medicine. J Regen Med 2016; 5:1. Sandeep Shrivastava, Chandrashekar Mahakalkar et al Platelet Rich Plasma as a for Diabetic Ulcer. J.Tissue Sci Eng 2016; 7:186.

- Mohammadi R, Mehrtash M, Mehrtash M, Hassani N, Hassanpour A. Effect of Platelet Rich Plasma Combined with Chitosan Biodegradable Film on Full-Thickness Wound Healing in Rat Model. Bull Emerg Trauma. 2016;4(1):29–37.

- Manish Suthar, Saniya Gupta et al Treatment of chronic non-healing ulcers

- using autologous platelet rich plasma: a case series J Biomed Sci. 2017; 24.

- Shrivastava S, Naik S, Patil B, Kharabe P, Gupta A, et al. Bio Technological Intervention with Platelet Rich Plasma for Assisted Regeneration of Sole. J Tissue Sci Eng 2017; 8: 206.

- Mahakalkar C, Shrivastava S, Gupta A, Naik S, Kaple M, et al Bio-Engineering of Wounds by PRP Led Regeneration. J Tissue Sci Eng 2017; 8: 208.

PRP & Cartilage & Tendon Regeneration

- Yang SY, Ahn ST, Rhie JW, et al.Platelet supernatant promotes proliferation of auricular chondrocytes and formation of chondrocyte mass. Ann Plast Surg 2000 44(4), 405–411.

- Gaissmaier C, Fritz J, Krackhardt T, et al. Effect of human platelet supernatant on proliferation and matrix synthesis of human articular chondrocytes in monolayer and three-dimensional alginate cultures. Biomaterials 2005; 26(14), 1953–1960.

- Akeda K, An HS, Okuma M, et al. Platelet-rich plasma stimulates porcine articular chondrocyte proliferation and matrix biosynthesis. Osteoarthritis Cartil 2006; 14(12), 1272–1280.

- Anitua E, Sanchez M, Nurden AT, et al. Platelet-released growth factors enhance the secretion of hyaluronic acid and induce hepatocyte growth factor production by synovial fibroblasts from arthritic patientsm. Rheumatology (Oxford) 2007; 46(12), 1769–1772.

- Anchez M, Anitua E, Azofra J, et al. Intra-articular injection of an autologous preparation rich in growth factors for the treatment of knee OA: a retrospective cohort study. Clin Exp Rheumatol 2008; 26, 910–913.

- Saito M, Takahashi KA, Arai Y, et al. Intra-articular administration of platelet-rich plasma with biodegradable gelatin hydrogel microspheres prevents osteoarthritis progression in the rabbit knee. Clin Exp Rheumatol 2009;(2), 201–207.

- Spreafico A, Chellini F, Frediani B, et al. Biochemical investigation of the effects of human platelet releasates on human articular chondrocytes. J Cell Biochem 2009;108(5), 1153–1165.

- Kon E, Buda R, Filardo G, et al.Platelet- rich plasma: intra-articular knee injections produced favorable results on degenerative cartilage lesions. Knee Surg Sports Traumatol Arthrosc 2010 18, 472–479.

- Bendinelli P, Matteucci E, Dogliotti G, et al. Molecular basis of anti-inflammatory action of platelet-rich plasma on human chondrocytes: mechanisms of NF-jB inhibition via HGF. J Cell Physiol 2010; 225(3), 757–766

- Van Buul GM, Koevoet WL, Kops N, et al.Platelet-rich plasma releasate inhibits inflammatory processes in osteoarthritic chondrocytes. Am J Sports Med 2011; 39(11), 2362–2370

- Wu CC, Chen WH, Zao B, et al. Regenerative potentials of platelet-rich plasma enhanced by collagen in retrieving pro-inflammatory cytokine-inhibited chondrogenesis. Biomaterials 2011 32(25), 5847–5854.

- Kon E, Mandelbaum B, Buda R, et al. Platelet-rich plasma intraarticular injection versus hyaluronic acid viscosupplementation as treatments for cartilage pathology: from early degeneration to osteoarthritis. Arthroscopy 2011; 27, 1490–1501.

- Dhillon M, Patel S, Bali K Platelet-rich plasma intra-articular knee injections for the treatment of degenerative cartilage lesions and osteoarthritis. Knee Surg Sports Traumatol Arthrosc 2011; 19, 863–864, author reply 865-866.

- Li M, Zhang C, Ai Z, et al. Therapeutic effectiveness of intra-knee-articular injection of platelet-rich plasma on knee articular cartilage degeneration. Zhongguo Xiu Fu Chong JianWai Ke Za Zhi 2011; 25(10), 1192–1196.

- Filardo G, Kon E, Buda R, et al. 2011 Platelet-rich plasma intra-articular knee injections for the treatment of degenerative cartilage lesions and osteoarthritis. Knee Surg Sports Traumatol Arthrosc 2011;19, 528–535.

- Dragoo JL, Braun HJ, Durham JL, et al. Comparison of the acute inflammatory response of two commercial platelet-rich plasma systems in healthy rabbit tendons. Am J Sports Med 2012 40(6), 1274–1281.

- Anitua E, Sanchez M, De la Fuente M, et al.Plasma rich in growth factors (PRGF-Endoret) stimulates tendon and synovial fibroblasts migration and improves the biological properties of hyaluronic acid. Knee Surg Sports Traumatol Arthrosc 2012; 20, 1657–1665.

- Lee HR, Park KM, Joung YK, et al. Platelet rich plasma loaded hydrogel scaffold enhances chondrogenic differentiation and maturation with up-regulation of CB1 and CB2. J Control Release1 2012; 59(3), 332–337.

- Park SI, Lee HR, Kim S, et al. Time sequential modulation in expression of growth factors from platelet-rich plasma (PRP) on the chondrocyte cultures. Mol Cell Biochem 2012 361(1–2), 9–17.

- Mishra A, Harmon K, Woodall J, et al. Sports medicine applications of platelet rich plasma. Curr Pharm Biotechnol 2012; 13, 1185–1195.

- DeLong JM, Russell RP, Mazzocca AD Platelet-rich plasma: the PAW classification system. J Arthrosc Relat Surg 2012 28, 998–1009.

- Sanchez M, Fiz N, Azofra J, et al.A randomized clinical trial evaluating plasma rich in growth factors (PRGF-Endoret) versus hyaluronic acid in the short-term treatment of symptomatic knee osteoarthritis. Arthroscopy 2012;28(8), 1070–1078

- Sanchez M, Guadilla J, Fiz N, et al.Ultrasound-guided platelet-rich plasma injections for the treatment of osteoarthritis of the hip. Rheumatology 2012 51, 144–150.

- Filardo G, Kon E, Pereira Ruiz MT, et al. Platelet-rich plasma intra-articular injections for cartilage degeneration and osteoarthritis: single- versus double- spinning approach. Knee Surg Sports Traumatol Arthrosc 2012; 20(10), 2082–2091.

- Spakova T, Rosocha J, Lacko M, et al. Treatment of knee joint osteoarthritis with autologous platelet-rich plasma in comparison with hyaluronic acid. Am J Phys Med Rehabil 2012; 91, 411–417.

- Cerza F, Carnì S, Carcangiu A, et al. Comparison between hyaluronic acid and platelet-rich plasma, intra-articular infiltration in the treatment of gonarthrosis. Am J Sports Med 2012 40, 2822–2827.

- Mei-Dan O, Carmont MR, Laver L, et al. Platelet-rich plasma or hyaluronate in the management of osteochondral lesions of the talus. Am J Sports Med 2012 40(3), 534–541.

- Say F, Gürler D, Yener K, et al. Platelet-rich plasma injection is more effective than hyaluronic acid in the treatment of knee osteoarthritis. Acta Chir Ortho Traumatol Cech 2013; 80(4), 278–283.

- Pereira RC, Scaranari M, Benelli R, et al. Dual effect of platelet lysate on human articular cartilage: a maintenance of chondrogenic potential and a transient proinflammatory activity followed by an inflammation resolution. Tissue Eng Part A 2013; 19(11–12), 1476–1488

- Yin Z, Yang X, Jiang Y, et al.Platelet-rich plasma combined with agarose as a bioactive scaffold to enhance cartilage repair: an in vitro study. J Biomater Appl 2013;28(7), 1039–1050.

- Hart R, Safi A, Komázk M, et al. Platelet-rich plasma in patients with tibiofemoral cartilage degeneration. Arch Orthop Trauma Surg 2013; 133(9), 1295–1301.

- Patel S, Dhillon MS, Aggarwal S, et al. Treatment with platelet-rich plasma is more effective than placebo for knee osteoarthritis: a prospective, double-blind, randomized trial. Am J Sports Med 2013; 41, 356–364.

- Kutlu B, Aydın RST, Akman AC, et al. Platelet-rich plasma-loaded chitosan scaffolds: preparation and growth factor release kinetics. J Biomed Materials Res Part B: Applied Biomaterials 2013; 101(1), 28–35.

- Battaglia M, Guaraldi F, Vannini F, et al. Efficacy of ultrasound-guided intra-articular injections of platelet-rich plasma versus hyaluronic acid for hip osteoarthritis. Orthopedics 2013; 36(12), e1501–e1508.

- Sundman EA, Cole BJ, Karas V, et al. The anti-inflammatory and matrix restorative mechanisms of platelet-rich plasma in osteoarthritis. Am J Sports Med 2014; 42(1), 35–41.

- Braun HJ, Kim HJ, Chu CR, et al. The effect of platelet-rich plasma formulations and blood products on human synoviocytes: implications for intra-articular injury and therapy. Am J Sports Med 2014; 42(5), 1204–1210.

- Patel S, Dhillon MS The anti-inflammatory and matrix restorative mechanisms of platelet-rich plasma in osteoarthritis: letter to the editor. Am J Sports Med2014 30, 42.

- Magalon J, Bausset O, Serratrice N, et al. Characterization and comparison of 5 platelet-rich plasma preparations in a single-donor model. Arthroscopy 2014 30(5), 629–638.

- Cavallo C, Filardo G, Mariani E, et al Comparison of platelet rich plasma formulations for cartilage healing: an in vitro study. J Bone Joint Surg (Am) 2014; 96(5), 5423–5429.

- Roffi A, Filardo G, Assirelli E, et al. Does platelet-rich plasma freeze-thawing influence growth factor release and their effects on chondrocytes and synoviocytes? Biomed Res Int 2014, 692913.

- Andia I, Abate M Knee osteoarthritis: hyaluronic acid, platelet-rich plasma or both in association? Expert Opin Biol Ther 2014 14, 635–649.

- Görmeli G, Görmeli CA, Ataoglu B, et al. Multiple PRP injections are more effective than single injections and hyaluronic acid in knees with early osteoarthritis: a randomized, double-blind, placebo-controlled trial. Knee Surg Sports Traumatol Arthrosc, 2015 DOI: 10.1007/s00167-015-3705-6.

- Filardo G, Di Matteo B, Martino Di, et al. Platelet-rich plasma intra-articular knee injections show no superiority versus visco-supplementation: a randomized controlled trial. Am J Sports Med 2015; 43(7), 1575–1582

- Hassan AS, El-Shafey AM, Ahmed HS, et al. Effectiveness of the intra-articular injection of platelet rich plasma in the treatment of patients with primary knee osteoarthritis. Egypt Rheumatol 2015 37(3), 119–124.

- Gobbi A, Lad D, Karnatzikos G The effects of repeated intra-articular PRP injections on clinical outcomes of early osteoarthritis of the knee. Knee Surg Sports Traumatol Arthrosc 2015 23(8), 2170–2177.

- Sánchez M, Fiz N, Guadilla J, et al. Intraosseous infiltration of platelet-rich plasma for severe knee osteoarthritis. Arthrosc Tech 2015 3(6), e713–e717.

- Riboh JC, Saltzman BM, Yanke AB, et al. Effect of leukocyte concentration on the efficacy of platelet-rich plasma in the treatment of knee osteoarthritis. Am J Sports Med 2016 (3), 792–800.

- Paterson KL, Nicholls M, Bennell KL, et al. () Intra-articular injection of photo-activated platelet-rich plasma in patients with knee osteoarthritis: a double-blind, randomized controlled pilot study. BMC Musculoskelet Disord 2016; 17, 67.

- Dallari D, Stagni C, Rani N, et al. Ultrasound-guided injection of platelet-rich plasma and hyaluronic acid, separately and in combination, for hip osteoarthritis: a randomized controlled study. Am J Sports Med 2016 44(3), 664–671.

- Lana JF, Weglein A, Sampson S, et al. Randomized controlled trial comparing hyaluronic acid, platelet-rich plasma and the combination of both in the treatment of mild and moderate osteoarthritis of the knee. J Stem Cells Regen Med 2016 12(2), 69–78.

PRP and Fracture Impairments

- Canalis E, McCarthy TL, Centrella M. Effects of platelet-derived growth factor on bone formation in vitro. J Cell Physiol 1989; 140:530-7.

- Weibrich G, Hansen T, Kleis W, Buch R, Hitzler WE. Effect of platelet concentration in platelet-rich plasma on peri-implant bone regeneration. Bone 2004; 34:665-71.

- Zimmermann G, Henle P, Küsswetter M, Moghaddam A, Wentzensen A, Richter W, et al. TGF-beta1 as a marker of delayed fracture healing. Bone 2005;36:779-85.

- Aghaloo TL, Moy PK, Freymiller EG. Investigation of platelet-rich plasma in rabbit cranial defects: A pilot study. J Oral Maxillofac Surg. 2002;60(10):1176–81.

- Okuda K, Tai H, Tanabe K, et al Platelet-rich plasma combined with a porous hydroxyapatite graft for the treatment of intrabony periodontal defects in humans: a comparative controlled clinical study. J Periodontol 2005; 76:890–898.

- Gerard D, Carlson ER, Gotcher JE, Jacobs M. Effects of platelet-rich plasma at the cellular level on healing of autologous bone-grafted mandibular defects in dogs. J Oral Maxillofac Surg. 2007;65(4):721–7.

- Galasso O, Mariconda M, Romano G, Capuano N, Romano L, Ianno B, et al. Expandable intramedullary nailing and platelet rich plasma to treat long bone non-unions. J Orthop Traumatol. 2008;9(3):129–34.

- Calori G, Tagliabue L, Gala L, d'Imporzano M, Peretti G, Albisetti W. Application of rhBMP-7 and platelet-rich plasma in the treatment of long bone non-unions: a prospective randomised clinical study on 120 patients. Injury. 2008;39(12):1391–402.

- Hakimi M, Jungbluth P, Sager M, Betsch M, Herten M, Becker J, et al. Combined use of platelet-rich plasma and autologous bone grafts in the treatment of long bone defects in mini-pigs. Injury. 2010;41(7):717–23.

- Sun Y, Feng Y, Zhang CQ, Chen SB, Cheng XG. The regenerative effect of platelet-rich plasma on healing in large osteochondral defects. Int Orthop. 2010;34(4):589–97.

- Kanthan SR, Kavitha G, Addi S, Choon DS, Kamarul T. Platelet-rich plasma (PRP) enhances bone healing in non-united critical-sized defects: a preliminary study involving rabbit models. Injury. 2011;42(8):782–9.

- Hakimi M, Jungbluth P, Thelen S, Betsch M, Linhart W, Flohe S, et al. Platelet-rich plasma combined with autologous cancellous bone: An alternative therapy for persistent non-union? Unfallchirurg. 2011;114(11):998–1006.

- Broggini N, Hofstetter W, Hunziker E, Bosshardt DD, Bornstein MM, Seto I, et al. The influence of PRP on early bone formation in membrane protected defects A histological and histomorphometric study in the rabbit calvaria. Clin Implant Dent Relat Res. 2011;13(1):1–12

- Liu HY, Wu AT, Tsai CY, Chou KR, Zeng R, Wang MF, et al. The balance between adipogenesis and osteogenesis in bone regeneration by platelet-rich plasma for age-related osteoporosis. Biomaterials 2011; 32:6773-80.

- Griffin XL, Wallace D, Parsons N, Costa ML. Platelet rich therapies for long bone healing in adults. Cochrane Database Syst Rev 2012; 7:CD009496.

- Roffi A, Filardo G, Kon E, Marcacci M. Does PRP enhance bone integration with grafts, graft substitutes, or implants? A systematic review. BMC Musculoskelet Disord. 2013; 14:330.

- Chen L, Yang X, Huang G, Song D, Ye XS, Xu H, et al. Platelet-rich plasma promotes healing of osteoporotic fractures. Orthopedics 2013;36:e687-94.

- Memeo A, Verdoni F, De Bartolomeo O, Albisetti W, Pedretti L. A new way to treat forearm post-traumatic non-union in young patients with intramedullary nailing and platelet-rich plasma. Injury. 2014;45(2):418–23.

- Say F, Turkeli E, Bulbul M. Is platelet-rich plasma injection an effective choice in cases of non-union? Acta Chir Orthop Traumatol Cech. 2014;81(5):340–5.

- Lee DH, Ryu KJ, Kim JW, Kang KC, Choi YR. Bone marrow aspirate concentrate and platelet-rich plasma enhanced bone healing in distraction osteogenesis of the tibia. Clin Orthop Relat Res. 2014;472(12):3789–97.

- Brossi PM, Moreira JJ, Machado TS, Baccarin RY. Platelet-rich plasma in orthopedic therapy: a comparative systematic review of clinical and experimental data in equine and human musculoskeletal lesions. BMC Vet Res. 2015; 11:98.

- Malhotra R, Kumar V, Garg B, Singh R, Jain V, Coshic P, et al. Role of autologous platelet-rich plasma in treatment of long-bone nonunions: a prospective study. Musculoskelet Surg. 2015;99(3):243–8.

- Samy AM. The role of platelet rich plasma in management of fracture neck femur: new insights. Int Orthop. 2016;40(5):1019–24.

- Singh A, Ali S, Srivastava RN. Platelet-rich plasma in osteoporotic fractures: A review of literature. J Orthop Traumatol Rehabil [serial online] 2014 [cited 2019 Sep 12];7: 123-38.

PRP in Infertility

A. Endometrium Regeneration

- Gleicher N, Kim A, Michaeli T, et al. A pilot cohort study of granulocyte colony-stimulating factor in the treatment of unresponsive thin endometrium resistant to standard therapies. Hum Reprod. 2013;28(1):172–177.

- Kunicki M, Aukaszuk K, Woclawek-Potocka I, et al. Evaluation of granulocyte colony-stimulating factor effects on treatment-resistant thin endometrium in women undergoing in vitro fertilization. BioMed Res Int. 2014; 2014:913235.

- Eftekhar M, Sayadi M, Arabjahvani F. Transvaginal perfusion of G-CSF for infertile women with thin endometrium in frozen ET program: a non-randomized clinical trial. Iran J Reprod Med. 2014;12(10):661–666.

- Yajie Chang, Jingjie Li, Yuqing Chen, Lina Wei, Xing Yang, Yanan Shi, Xiaoyan Liang

- Autologous platelet-rich plasma promotes endometrial growth and improves pregnancy outcome during in vitro fertilization Int J Clin Exp Med. 2015; 8(1): 1286–1290.

- Li Y, Pan P, Chen X, et al. Granulocyte colony-stimulating factor administration for infertile women with thin endometrium in frozen embryo transfer program. Reprod Sci. 2014; 21:381–385.

- Sara Pedri,1 Daniela Lico,1 Annalisa Di Cello,1 Pietro D'Alessandro,1 Alberto Vaiarelli,2 Erminia Alviggi,3 Alberto Vincenzo Filardo,4 Antonio Gallucci,5 Andrea Dominijanni,6 Fulvio Zullo,1 and Roberta Venturella; Thin endometrium in patient undergoing Assisted Reproductive Technology: pathogenesis and treatment 2016 January-February; 3(1): 1–11. ISSN: 2385-2836

B. Ovarian Rejuvenation

- Pantos K, Nitsos N, Kokkali G, Vaxevanoglou T, Markomichali C, Pantou A, Grammatis M, Lazaros L, Sfakianoudis K. Ovarian rejuvenation and folliculogenesis reactivation in peri-menopausal women after autologous platelet-rich plasma treatment. InProceedings of the 32nd Annual Meeting of ESHRE 2016 Jul 1 (pp. 3-6).

- Ljubić A, Abazović D, Vučetić D, Ljubić D, Pejović T, Božanović T. Case Report Autologous ovarian in vitro activation with ultrasound-guided orthotopic re-transplantation. Am J Clin Exp Obstet Gynecol. 2017;4(5):51-7.

- Kothari K. Role of platelet-rich plasma: The current trend and evidence. Indian Journal of Pain. 2017 Jan 1;31(1):1.

- Sills ES, Rickers NS, Li X, Palermo GD. First data on in vitro fertilization and blastocyst formation after intraovarian injection of calcium gluconate-activated autologous platelet rich plasma. Gynecological Endocrinology. 2018 Sep 2;34(9):756-60

About Authors

Dr. Sandeep Shrivastava, MBBS, MS, DNB, Ph.D.

An Eminent Orthopaedic Surgeon and Medical Educationist.

He has worked on PRP treatment of wounds for more than a decade developing the STARS therapy.

He is Ex-Dean of Jawaharlal Nehru Medical College, Wardha, India.

He holds expertise in Limb Lengthening and Reconstruction.

Currently he is Chief Executive Officer (Hospitals); Director-Professor – Orthopaedics and Hon. Director for Centre of Regenerative Medicine (a Centre for Excellence) at Datta Meghe Institute of Medical Sciences, Sawangi, Wardha. India

Dr. Deepti Shrivastava, MBBS, MD, Ph.D

An Eminent Obstetrician and Gynecologist.

She has been working with PRP in various aspects of Infertility including for Endometrial and Follicular Regenerations.

She is a Reproductive Medicine Expert.

She is Director of Wardha Test-tube Centre (IVF Centre of DMIMS) and

Professor of Obstetrics and Gynaecology at JNMC, Datta Meghe Institute of Medical Sciences (DU), Sawangi, Wardha, India.

BACK PAGE

Include the Exclusive:

ATLAS ON STARS Therapy.

(Sandeep's Technique for Assisted Regeneration of Skin)*

The *Game Changer* Regenerative Care for Wounds.

Step into the world of next generation health care solutions

doing away with Surgery, Drugs, and Hospitalizations.

A simple technique for Complex Wounds which can be practiced by all Health Care providers – Experts, Doctors, Physician Assistants and Nurses

It has opened up a very exciting possibility for tissue preservation & regeneration in complex acute, postoperative, burst- abdomen, chronic non-healing, infected, necrotic & gangrenes wounds.

* Copyrighted under Indian Laws.